The Seven Ages of Death

By the same author

Unnatural Causes

The Seven Ages of Death

A Forensic Pathologist's Journey Through Life

DR RICHARD SHEPHERD

MICHAEL 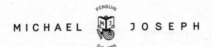 JOSEPH

MICHAEL JOSEPH

UK | USA | Canada | Ireland | Australia
India | New Zealand | South Africa

Michael Joseph is part of the Penguin Random House group of companies
whose addresses can be found at global.penguinrandomhouse.com

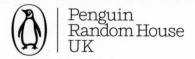

First published by Michael Joseph 2021
001

Set in 13.5/16pt Garamond MT Std
Typeset by Jouve (UK), Milton Keynes
Printed and bound in Great Britain by Clays Ltd, Elcograf S.p.A.

The authorized representative in the EEA is Penguin Random House Ireland,
Morrison Chambers, 32 Nassau Street, Dublin D02 YH68

A CIP catalogue record for this book is available from the British Library

HB ISBN: 978–0–241–47203–3
OM ISBN: 978–0–241–47204–0

www.greenpenguin.co.uk

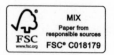

To my wonderful family for all the happiness
that you have given me, and especially to my wife, Linda,
who undoubtedly is my saviour in so many ways.

Author's Note

In my first book, *Unnatural Causes*, I explained how difficult it had been for me to change names and identifying details of the cases I discussed. Throughout my working life I have strived for accuracy – but at the same time, I have tried to alleviate the suffering of the bereaved. It was a hard decision, but I finally made those changes because I would not want any reader to recognize a relative in print and perhaps unexpectedly revisit their darkest days. The same is true of this book. The names of those whose stories are too well known to disguise are given. In all other cases I have changed personal details to preserve confidentiality while maintaining relevant facts. It must also be acknowledged that this is a book about death. It contains sensitive but unflinching descriptions of those who have died from both natural and unnatural causes, from infants to the very old. I sincerely hope that you do not find this upsetting.

All the world's a stage,
And all the men and women merely players:
They have their exits and their entrances;
And one man in his time plays many parts,
His acts being seven ages. At first the infant,
Mewling and puking in the nurse's arms;
And then the whining school-boy, with his satchel
And shining morning face, creeping like snail
Unwillingly to school: And then the lover;
Sighing like furnace, with a woeful ballad
Made to his mistress' eyebrow: Then a soldier,
Full of strange oaths, and bearded like the pard,
Jealous in honour, sudden and quick in quarrel,
Seeking the bubble reputation
Even in the cannon's mouth. And then the justice;
In fair round belly with good capon lin'd,
With eyes severe and beard of formal cut,
Full of wise saws and modern instances;
And so he plays his part: The sixth age shifts
Into the lean and slipper'd pantaloon;
With spectacles on nose and pouch on side;
His youthful hose, well sav'd, a world too wide
For his shrunk shank; and his big manly voice,
Turning again toward childish treble, pipes
And whistles in his sound: Last scene of all,
That ends this strange eventful history,
Is second childishness and mere oblivion;
Sans teeth, sans eyes, sans taste, sans everything.

– *As You Like It*, Act 2, Scene 7, William Shakespeare

Prologue

As my father lay dying, I took his hand gently and squeezed it. How thin his busy fingers had become, and how still now. And how strange it felt to touch him in this way. He had been both parents to me since my mother's death when I was nine and, although I loved him deeply and somehow used to curl on his lap as a leggy child, I would not say that we were a physically demonstrative family. Now, I was reminded of my childhood, feeling his soft, warm hand in mine.

There was a significant divide between our post-war generation and our fathers'. Brought up by people who were young in Victoria's reign, impacted by the catastrophe that was the First World War, youthful in the midst of a global depression, active in the Second World War; well, of course they were different from boomers like us, the generation that has had it all.

I watched his body. He was propped up on the pillows. His eyes were closed. His chest rose and fell. Slowly, rhythmically. I knew that soon the rhythm would stop. I thought of the way he had conducted himself throughout his life, how all his behaviour had shown his humanity and respect for others. His quiet life, his small triumphs. His hobbies. The way he recorded music from the radio and then filed the cassettes endearingly in his orderly, accountant's fashion. The undemonstrative but undoubted love of his Sunday phone calls and weekly family newsletters once we had left home. The unbearable absence we were approaching.

I said goodbye. I told him what a wonderful father he had

been and how proud my long-dead mother would have been of him for the great care he had shown us. But I did not say I loved him. He knew that, and his generation was more comfortable knowing it than hearing it. I drove away from the hospice sure that I would not see him again. It was a bright September day. I noticed Devon's autumnal beauty even through my tears. I let them fall. That is what we do when death takes one we love. We cry and cry. What else can we do?

I was back in London, deep in court cases and post-mortems, when my brother arrived in Devon to take up the bedside vigil. Later that week, when the phone rang, somehow I knew who it would be and what news that voice would bring.

It was a peaceful death. The simple closing of a life. Of course, it was well managed by the hospice staff. There was no pain and my brother was at his side. My father had seen all of us in the last few days and our presence had reassured him – of our love and of our stable lives, which he had done so much to establish. He could take the final step of life's journey without anxiety about whatever would happen in the world when he left it. He was an atheist, but he always believed, hoped, that he would join my mother one day. And he accepted that this was his time to die. He slipped peacefully away.

After the call, I sat at my desk. A new numbness; mental, physical.

A file lay open in front of me. It was a murder file. Its pictures, now scattered across my desk, showed me a very different end of life. It is my profession to examine the deceased and, for the vast majority of those I encounter, death has come too soon and seldom calmly. How easy it is for me to forget that my father's sweet departure is the norm.

The day after his funeral, I was back at work. Dealing with those other kinds of death.

At first the infant,
Mewling and puking in the nurse's arms;

I

Schoolbooks lost, one trainer under the kitchen table, the kids singing the comic song which was even now blaring from radios all over Britain, bickering over the words, missing the right notes but rising to the inevitable chorus, sandwiches half made, me panicking over the time. It was Monday morning.

I dropped the children off at school five minutes later than usual. They bounced through the gates. I watched them. I loved the new silence in the car and missed their noise at the same time. How fast children grow; it would be new coats next winter. My daughter turned back suddenly. She was laughing at something, perhaps even still singing. When she saw that I had not moved, she immediately waved her hand with an intensity and passion that only children can muster for a handwave. My son saw her, turned and treated me to a lop-sided grin. I lifted an arm to wave, but they were gone. A bell was ringing somewhere.

And so, to work. I turned on the car radio and here was their favourite song again. Oh no. But I didn't switch it off. Although I had heard it at least ten times already this morning, now it made me smile. The way my children pulled ridiculous faces as they sang it.

I reached the mortuary and saw a couple of police cars were there already. It was time to enter my other world.

Soon, a group of detectives and the coroner's officer were hovering in their scrubs outside the post-mortem room, their mortuary wellies still gleaming from the footbath. They weren't really waiting for me, they just didn't want to go in. And, although death is my life, neither did I. Everyone hates that moment when they see the baby.

We present a benign world to the young by dressing them in gentle, pastel colours. And we protect them from life's harshness and its cold by surrounding them with softness: the woolly blankets, the fuzzy toys, the cosy clothes. All that is stripped away here. So when we walked in to find the baby lying on a hard surface, dwarfed by the table, the trolleys, the fridges, when we saw rounded cheeks and tiny fingers in that stark, shiny, metallic place . . . well, for a moment even the prepared mind must go through contortions to rationalize this sight.

It lasted only a moment. Then the officers silently took their places around the trolley.

The detective inspector's eyes slid from the baby to the soft toy, which the staff had put to one side. A funerary offering, left by the boy's suffering parents as a friend to love and keep him safe in his new, strange place. No doubt more toys would be buried with him. Humans have made these offerings all through history, but a dog-eared teddy is more poignant than all the gold in Tutankhamun's tomb.

'You all right, boss?' said one of the detectives to the inspector. The corner of her mouth was twitching. She nodded.

'We're here to do a job for this baby, we're here in the spirit of compassion and scientific discovery,' I said. Using my firm voice. Hoping I sounded brisk enough to stop any tears that might threaten to leak over the pristine surfaces of the post-mortem room. Emotion is what we *don't* do in here. Or where would it end?

The inspector gulped. 'The parents . . .'

'The boss had a baby last year,' said her colleague. He was trying to excuse her great sadness, but it really needed no excuse.

'I've got two children and it's very hard not to think of them when I find a child in the post-mortem room,' I said. 'But your baby is safe and sound and the best thing we can do for the parents of er' – I shuffled through my notes – 'Fergusson, Fergusson Bell, is to find out why he died.'

The detective inspector nodded gravely and surveyed Fergusson's body.

He was six months old.

'Fat little cheeks,' the younger detective said.

'Yeah, chubby fellow.' The coroner's officer nodded. 'Just look at that tummy.'

'He's a good size for six months,' I agreed. 'But I think there may be some swelling in his arms and legs, and as for his abdomen . . .'

I placed a couple of fingers on his belly and tapped them. Everyone listened to the sound of a tiny drum. I moved and tapped again. And again. And once more. Always a drum.

'It's gas,' I said. 'Nothing solid. And now I look at his face, it's not quite right.'

'Why not, Doc?'

I didn't know exactly why not.

'May be swollen too.'

We photographed the baby then took off his clothes, the ones which hadn't already been removed by the paramedics who had tried to revive him. We did this carefully: parents often ask for the return of the clothes their child died in.

Then I took off his nappy.

'My God!' the super gasped.

'Will you look at that!' the coroner's officer said.

'Outrageous!' the detective muttered.

I have exposed a lot of hideous wounds to a lot of police officers over the years – wounds inflicted by all manner of weapons, caused for all manner of reasons, from blind passion to genuine error . . . but they have seldom been received with such an outcry. And what had prompted that response today?

Nappy rash.

It spread from the baby's belly to his thighs and much of it was raw and red and bleeding. The photographer took pictures in silence. The officers, however, could not stop talking.

'All you have to do is put on the cream,' the inspector said. 'Why couldn't anyone be bothered to do that?'

'No excuse,' the coroner's officer agreed.

'I mean, it's so easy. It costs so little . . . and it clears up in no time.'

'Notes say the kid was crying a lot before he died . . .' reported the detective.

'How long before he died?' I asked.

'Er . . . three weeks.'

'Three weeks!' the inspector breathed. 'He cried for three weeks!'

I said: 'No one ever died of nappy rash. But it might explain the gas in the bowel. If he was in pain and crying all the time, he'd be off his food and swallowing a lot of air . . . on the other hand, I may find some other reason he's full of gas.'

The detective said: 'Well, the hospital suggested SIDS for cause of death.'

Maybe it was. Children are more likely to die suddenly, for no apparent reason, in neglectful homes, and if this nappy rash said anything to me, it said neglect. The state of a nappy can be a great indicator: distressingly, I have even found the paper liner in the bowels of small children who were so hungry that they had eaten their own nappies.

There are many reasons for neglect, some of them complex. I wished I'd been given a bit more information about this case, been told something about the parents or the circumstances but, as usual at this stage, there was very little context.

'Did you go to the home?' I asked the detective.

'Yeah, my most unfavourite job.'

'And?'

'And nothing. Nice little semi. Not badly off. Middle-class neighbourhood.'

'But was the house chaotic?' Not that ours had been entirely tidy when we had babies. But the homes of heavy drinkers, for instance, have a distinctive chaos. The dusty exercise equipment vying for space with discarded baby toys, bags of nappies, piles of laundry and many, many bottles.

'Nope. Very tidy.'

'No drink, no drugs?'

'No evidence of that and, frankly, I doubt it. Baby stopped crying and they put him to bed, mother went in an hour later and found him dead. Called an ambulance but it was too late. That's all we've got, really.'

'Do the parents have jobs?'

'Yeah . . . she's a secretary or administrator or something and he's . . . I think he's a doctor.'

'A doctor?' the inspector said. 'A *doctor*! How could he let his kid have nappy rash like that!'

'Oh, I don't think doctors always make the best parents,' I said, trying not to think too hard about that as I examined Fergusson.

9

'Didn't like the father when I interviewed him,' said the detective. 'I'd say he was . . . hostile.'

'Means nothing,' the coroner's officer said. 'People behave in strange ways when they've had a tragedy, and then the police come round asking them questions which make them feel it's all their fault.'

The detective looked back at him squarely.

'Sometimes,' he said, 'it is their fault.'

I was looking at Fergusson carefully for signs of ill treatment as well as further neglect, but there were none. No bruises, no burns, no cuts or scratches, just evidence of the paramedics' efforts. Apart from the nappy rash and bloated abdomen, there was only one other noteworthy feature of his body. His pallor. People describe Caucasian faces, perhaps after a shock, as a 'deathly white', but death does not necessarily make people much paler than they are in life. Fergusson, however, was distinctly pallid.

When the time came to cut open the body, the room became very silent and the inspector looked away. As usual, I talked them through the biology. The human body is truly fascinating if you can put your feelings of revulsion to one side. I try to persuade horrified observers of this. Not always successfully.

I made the incision we use specifically for babies and small children: instead of the usual Y-shape, we use a T-shape, the top line passing horizontally across the front of the chest to keep the neck well clear of any stitches. All our incisions are made to cause minimum pain to relatives who ask to see the body. So, never avoid a body after a post-mortem. The loved one you remember will be there waiting for you.

Now I made the cut so swiftly that the inspector barely had time to draw breath. Then I exposed the lungs. Here I found fluid, filling a good proportion of the chest cavity. There was so much that one lung had partially collapsed. I took a sample.

'Is that how he died?' The detective inspector was already starting to look more fascinated than revolted. 'The collapsed lung?'

'I doubt it. That probably happened because there simply wasn't room for the lung in his chest with all this fluid. And the fluid only tells us his heart gradually failed. But not why.'

'Gradually? That means it can't be SIDS, then,' the detective said. The others nodded.

'Too soon to be sure,' I told him. In fact, with Sudden Infant Death Syndrome, we can never be sure. We can only rule out everything else.

I opened the rest of the body and, glancing at the inspector, saw that she had shut her eyes.

'Try to see this small body for the miracle it is,' I said.

Fergusson had died at six months for some reason we had yet to understand, but every child born, even one who lives such a short time, is one of nature's dazzling achievements. Just getting on to the starting blocks is hazardous enough. Long before our lives begin, our parents' sperm or eggs are created from precursor cells by an extraordinary process called meiosis. Why is it extraordinary? Because sperm and egg cells aren't simply replicas of parents' cells. No, meiosis is designed to halve the chromosomes in sperm and egg cells so that the two can combine to make, hopefully, one whole. And meiosis involves an extra, rather dangerous process, the crossover stage. During this, chromosomes which have been paired together now mix up their DNA. The artist has carefully been dabbing each separate colour on to the canvas. Now the brush goes on the palette and is whirled around to create completely new colours. That's the unique part. Result: the DNA in a woman's eggs isn't exactly like her mother's. Generational differences have been established long before DNA gets mixed up for the final time – when sperm and egg eventually meet.

But whirling a brush around in a lot of colours is potentially messy as well as beautiful, so the vital crossover stage is also a key moment for chromosomal abnormalities to occur. And in females this event, which will so affect a future child, actually happens long before that child is conceived. In fact, the crossover happens while the mother-to-be is still in her own mother's womb, so during the very early weeks of the grandmother's pregnancy. It can be hard to believe that events in Grandma's life can so influence the ovaries of the baby in her womb. There is much resulting debate about the extent to which meiosis is affected by environmental and physical factors . . . but if someone suggests that, for instance, the Chernobyl disaster in 1986 may still be having an impact two generations on, well, this may not be an idea to dismiss.

Once the sperm fertilizes the egg, something takes place which is, metabolically speaking, like a nuclear explosion. The moment of conception – that is, when the two 'half' DNAs from each parent combine – starts a sprint to divide and develop which really is spectacular. We are now into mitosis, when cells divide to produce exact replicas of themselves, rather than the mix-up that goes into the production of sperm and egg.

But this extraordinary speed means that mitosis is another danger area, when mistakes can occur which end life long before birth.

Congenital conditions – disorders a baby is born with – have many causes.

First, there are external factors. These may be physical, like a lack of amniotic fluid to protect the developing baby so parts of the body are squished and stay squished. Or the mother (perhaps even the grandmother) may be exposed to such dangers as radiation or mercury, or she herself may expose her baby to dangers like alcohol. Viruses are another major external threat. For instance, the 1918 Spanish 'flu pandemic killed 50 to 100 million people worldwide and particularly affected the young. In the USA, about a third of women who were pregnant or of childbearing age became infected. Long-term health studies in the United States of the children who were in utero when their mothers contracted the 'flu have concluded that these children may have faced health consequences many years later. Where mothers caught 'flu very early in their pregnancy, their children showed a greater tendency later on to diabetes. Contracting 'flu in early to mid-pregnancy significantly increased the child's chances of developing heart disease in later life, even in old age. And 'flu in the final months of pregnancy meant that the child might be more susceptible to kidney disorders on reaching late adulthood.

The 'flu virus is assumed to have placed the foetus under stress, and one theory – one of many – is that under such stress the blood supply switches from vital organs to the brain of the foetus in order to protect it. This ensures survival but may pre-programme certain organs for failure fifty, sixty or more years later. Different organs, of course, are developing at different times in the pregnancy, hence the relevance of the trimester in which the mother caught 'flu.

You might now be concerned that the world's most recent pandemic may have similar effects. But perhaps Covid-19 will not at all affect the long-term health of babies conceived and carried at this time: 'flu greatly affected the young whereas, in general, Covid has targeted the old. Long-term studies will answer this question, studies I will unfortunately not be around to read.

The second, equally unlucky, cause of congenital disorders is inherited familial genes. The disorders they carry may not be discernible at birth because the effects of some genes lie hidden for years before causing illness or death. Most show in the first few years of life, but Huntington's Chorea is one that is dormant for forty, fifty, even sixty years.

Genetic mistakes are the third and most common cause of congenital problems. They can happen during the creation of sperm (a process which may have taken place just a few weeks ago) or during the creation of eggs (a process from a more distant past, in the grandmother's womb). Or things may have gone wrong during the intense rate of cell multiplication after conception. In fact, if there are mistakes during pregnancy, the most likely time for these errors to occur is during the first four weeks. The organs, such as they are, lie so close together and their development is so interdependent that an error at this stage is often fatal. And even if there is no miscarriage and the foetus survives until birth, these early mistakes may cause such gross defects of the brain or heart that the baby lives only a short time.

In contrast, errors at a late stage of pregnancy can produce congenital defects which are not immediately obvious and may never be detected. I have occasionally stumbled across congenital heart defects at the post-mortem of an elderly person which did not cause death or illness and which I am sure no one ever knew about.

A baby's safe arrival in this world does not mark the end of a very hazardous journey. Those who survive birth still have what may well be the most dangerous year of their life directly ahead of them. The risk of death then drops significantly and we don't come close again to the hazards of that first year until we are fifty-five. At this point, destructive habits, illnesses related to ageing, accidents – perhaps resulting from a failure to recognize age's diminution of capabilities, unnatural occurrences like pollution or a murderous spouse, even those unnoticed congenital defects – all start to take their toll.

When I looked at Fergusson Bell, I could see there was neglect here – although, curiously, it was evidenced only in his nappy rash. But when I looked at his pallor and swollen abdomen, I was fairly sure that here was a congenital problem. Could it have been caused by a virus his mother had caught? Some errant gene? Or perhaps a mistake that had occurred as his cells multiplied in the womb? Whatever it was, it had revealed itself at an age when most babies are being weaned.

Fergusson's bowel was distended. The fluid which had caused one lung to collapse had left all his tissues saturated like a face cloth: this was certainly indicative of osmotic changes during heart failure as he died, so perhaps there was a congenital heart defect.

But if not his heart, then what?

Despite the effects of the fluid, the interior of his body looked faultless. A stunning landscape that had been created in nine months but perfected over millennia. It delights me, each time I see it, and that is many thousands of times, to note how the organs are nestled in the right cavity in the right way, each designed for the correct performance of their contribution to the living body.

In babies, the most beautiful organ is the brain. It is

perfectly formed but not yet firmed. At first it is glimpsed only through the frosted-glass window of the meninges that covers it. Beneath that, the matter is a yellow grey, translucent in places, wrapped in a fascinating pattern of red blood vessels. It is covered by the cortical ribbon, which is the pale brown of fine leather but much thinner. This is sometimes compared to foil covering an Easter egg, but words like 'ribbon' and 'foil' glamorize its steadfast pilgrimage into the valleys and over the mountains of the brain's ancient geography.

Beneath the ribbon, a child's brain is soft and gelatinous, resembling a walnut in its outer shape but not in size, colour or consistency. Inside the walnut, a baby's brain is pale: it will reach white as it firms; in other words, as myelin continues to sheathe the nerve cells for the next twenty-five years. And deep, deep within this is more grey: the grey of the buried simian brain. Here is that part which our busy conscious minds forget, which continues to work when our more accessible functions let us down. The steady, unseen friend that keeps our heart beating, our lungs breathing, our immune system attacking invaders, our hormones balancing, our eyes blinking . . . this autonomic system is silent but perpetually busy.

Fergusson's brain had beauty and no apparent problems: in fact, all his organs looked healthy. Except, perhaps, for one. Was his liver too big? The liver is a large organ, and it seems particularly large in babies. It is earthy in colour, a deep red-brown, and lies at the top right of the abdomen but is so big that it stretches into the left side too. Something about the liver's deceptively haphazard position, the way it flops lazily across other organs, reminds me of a big cat lying in some chosen, sunny spot.

'This may be interesting . . .' I told the officers.

They craned their necks as I examined Fergusson's liver. I wasn't sure, not until I had cut into it and then rotated my scalpel under the mortuary lights – an old habit, that. But when the blade did not glimmer back at me as it should, I knew. Grease. Fergusson had a fatty liver.

I could exclude the commonest cause of an enlarged and fatty liver – heavy drinking. Drinking is an abuse of a spectacular organ, but the liver is forgiving. An older person's liver may be greasy after a good night out but should repair itself if its owner abstains for a while. When good nights out, lots of them, have become a lifestyle choice, the grease turns to butter. Think of the liver of a habitually heavy drinker as a lump of foie gras. By now it has become severely overloaded and the fat-logged cells are starting to collapse and die. They are replaced by connective tissue, and this process is known to most of us as scarring. Scarring blocks and distorts the blood supply, starving the remaining liver cells of oxygen. The result is further scarring: in fact, there is a tipping point for alcoholics where even abstinence cannot stop the advance of the progressive disease that is cirrhosis. And so, finally, we have a liver that is no longer bulging and buttery but more reminiscent of a pickled gherkin, small, misshapen, its surface crusty and pitted.

Fergusson's liver had a smooth beauty, but I did, in fact, test it for alcohol since it showed all the signs of an evening in the pub. Over the years these tests have shown that many a parent has quietened the baby in this way. But not Fergusson's. By now my suspicions were strengthening. The pallor, the swelling, the fatty liver: I was almost sure that he had been unlucky enough to inherit a faulty gene.

I looked up.

'I'll put my money on an inborn error of metabolism.'

The inspector blinked.

'What's that?'

'There are dozens of them. They're always inherited and they mean that the body can't metabolize something in the child's diet so it builds until it causes immense harm.'

'I've never heard of that,' said the coroner's officer.

'Is it like having a peanut allergy?' the detective asked.

'It's not an allergy but it's probably related to Fergusson's diet and it means that something wasn't working properly when he ate certain foods.'

'But he's only six months,' the inspector said. 'What could he be eating that . . . ?'

'I imagine the mother was just weaning him on to solids.'

The inspector wasn't satisfied.

'Then why wasn't she doing it gradually so she could work out what was bothering him?'

I got back to my work: there is so much to study and note about every unexplained death. But I knew that, since seeing the shocking nappy rash, the inspector was not going to feel kindly towards the parents. We needed more information – from the parents but also from my colleagues – because here was a case for specialists. Every inborn error of metabolism is rare, but there are a lot of them and so this is a very busy paediatric discipline.

Later, when the biochemistry results from the baby's blood and urine came back, I took them straight to a paediatrician. To identify the problem, we worked our way through most of the relevant specialists at my hospital: St George's, London.

Initially it seemed Fergusson had succumbed to a virus. Immunofluorescence for parvovirus was found in his liver, but the virologists' further studies led them to believe this must have been a false positive. As I'd suspected, we were soon back in genetic departments, surrounded by that burgeoning number of experts on inborn errors of metabolism.

There was very extensive testing and much discussion; in fact, it took about five months for all the experts to agree that Fergusson had suffered from an undiagnosed congenital metabolic weakness – which had indeed revealed itself only when he was given solid food. His body was unable to metabolize fructose, the natural sugar commonly found in fruit and that most common of substances, table sugar.

Fructose is a critical step in the metabolic chain that converts sugars to energy in order to power our cells. The body can make glycogen, the chemical which stores energy reserves – but the lack of enzymes means this cannot be broken down and the energy released. And so the liver can become as enlarged and fatty as that of a heavy drinker.

The metabolism expert expressed surprise that a baby in our medically advanced world could die of this rare disorder – because it could and should have been picked up and the child's diet adapted long before he was in any danger.

So what went wrong for Fergusson? A very unhappy conjunction of events. So unhappy that the inspector was keen to prosecute.

The parents were now questioned extensively. When I started reading the inspector's notes, I felt that here was a child who was greatly loved by parents who were doing what they believed to be the right thing for him. The father was not a doctor but a practitioner of alternative medicine and both he and the mother had a deep distrust of conventional doctors. So the child had not been seen by a professional of any kind since his birth: there had been no health visitor, no routine weighing, no checks and certainly no vaccinations.

Once the mother started to wean Fergusson, the parents had devised what they considered to be an entirely natural, suitable, safe and sustaining diet for him in line with their beliefs. There were molasses, cider vinegar, honey, some soya milk . . . plus fruit and vegetables. They had absolutely no way of knowing that their carefully thought-out diet would kill their son. Fergusson was unable to metabolize fruit and, very possibly, not the components of molasses, honey or soya milk either. By feeding him all this, they were – unwittingly – giving him terrible diarrhoea, which had caused the grotesque nappy rash. And they were also fatally impairing his liver function.

Alarmed by his constant crying, the father had eventually taken Fergusson to a colleague, a homeopath, who had advised them strongly to go to a GP. She noted the baby's very bad nappy rash and urged the use of a conventional cream to clear it rapidly. This consultation was extremely difficult as Fergusson screamed throughout and the father took his colleague's suggestions amiss. He angrily insisted that he did not believe in doctors of conventional medicine and that he would certainly not apply any over-the-counter remedy: he regarded this as suppressive and thought it would 'stop the rash from coming out'.

As I read these words, I felt my sympathy for the bereaved man begin to ebb a little. But could the rash really be as bad as I remembered? I pulled up the pictures that had been taken at the post-mortem and yes, it was extensive, raw and bloody. Two weeks after he had refused to follow his colleague's advice, the baby was dead. Of course, a hereditary condition, and not the rash, had killed him. However, I was sure that the inspector would think that when the child became so upset during weaning the parents were at the very least negligent in not seeing a doctor or even revising their chosen diet.

Her letter to me was measured: 'Maybe Mr Bell's deep-seated beliefs affected his judgement in the care of his son.' It is true that hereditary disorders of this kind are usually picked up and dealt with very quickly by a GP. Sometimes identification of the exact defect is delayed because there are many metabolic disorders, and most are rare. But, once identified, a simple adaptation in diet usually changes everything. As I had guessed, the inspector pointed this out and said she intended to take the case against Mr and Mrs Bell forward.

I was glad the Crown Prosecution Service did not agree with her. The Bells should, ideally, have consulted a doctor when they realized Fergusson was ill, but they were doing what was the best thing for their child, according to their own creed. They could not have known that Fergusson had a 1 in 10,000 or, some believe, a 1 in 100,000 disorder. I remained fairly sympathetic and expected to hear little more about the Bells. But I was to encounter them again and, by this time, their case had a strange resonance in my own life.

Unlike most doctors, my job is not primarily to prevent death but to explore it fully. A forensic pathologist is called when there has been a sudden or unexplained death. Sometimes to the scene itself, always to the body. I do perhaps have a special relationship with the dead. I don't share any of the fears or even repulsion which many people seem to feel at the prospect of encountering them. The dead cannot be hurt. And yet each body, whether life was ended by natural or unnatural causes, illustrates for me humanity's great vulnerability. The dead fill me with compassion. They lie naked and still, unable to defend themselves or offend others. Whatever may have been complex in life is now simple, whatever was secret is now laid bare, whatever mattered is now unimportant.

My fundamental question is: why did this person die? Discovering the truth can be a long journey for those involved, starting at the place the body was found, next in the post-mortem room and from there meandering through a range of experts – as well as doctors, these might include specialists in flies, pollen, blood spattering, criminal psychology and much more, onwards through forensic laboratories, where even minute quantities of DNA can now be analysed and ballistics reconstructed.

Sometimes, despite best efforts, truth is elusive and the death remains a mystery. Sometimes there are many truths to uncover. Where foul play is evident, the outcome is, we hope, a prosecution – or at least a fair courtroom trial. What, for me, started with a post-mortem, may end on the witness stand in court, where I can spend hours (sometimes days or even weeks) as my medical opinion is interpreted, reinterpreted and challenged by defence and prosecution.

So my work brings me into extremely close contact with the drowned, the decomposed, the burnt, the unlucky, the desperately unhappy, the murdered . . . I can be fascinated, perplexed or greatly sorrowful all in one day.

A means of escape is sometimes vital. I mean a way to forget and perhaps recover from the immense emotional burdens which the dead can unknowingly place on those who work with them – no matter how detached we try to be. And at that time of my life, holidays brought nurture. We had tried Greece, Turkey, the usual destinations which featured hot sand . . . but there was no place like home. Specifically, my parents-in-laws' home. This was a large house on the Isle of Man, surrounded by its own farmland, with stunning views of the sea as well as the storms that marched across it. There were beaches a-plenty, mountain and moorland walks ... but nothing compared to the welcome we received from my wife's parents, Austin and Maggie. I basked in their warmth, their delight at seeing us and spending time with our two children, their amazing ability to produce a delicious meal or a good malt whisky or a roaring fire before you'd even realized you wanted one.

There are just a few people who are truly life-enhancing, and Austin and Maggie were two of them. And, on the Isle of Man, for the first time, it occurred to me that examining the dead all day in a sterile post-mortem room and then returning to a house which functioned quietly around our quotidian routines might be a bit, well, bleak.

Austin and Maggie had an extremely active social life. When we stayed with them, we'd dress up for cocktails and go out and talk and laugh with their friends and then move on somewhere else for supper. This couldn't be more different from our home life. Two busy doctors had no time for dinner parties, let alone cocktails. We occasionally invited the neighbours for a meal, but watching Maggie and Austin in action simply showed me how poor a host I was and how inept a player in the welcoming game.

By complete coincidence, that year, my cousin Geoff had some financial business on the Isle of Man just when we were on our jolly, noisy Isle of Man holidays – and exactly at the time I was immersed in the Fergusson Bell case. He had a special link with that part of my childhood which pre-dated my mother's early death. His mother was my mother's sister and occasionally in my aunt's look or trick of speech I could, even in adulthood, be overwhelmed by a sense of familiarity. An aunt, sibling or cousin would do that to me, just occasionally: allow me to glimpse that very important person I had lost.

As if that link wasn't enough, Geoff and I had been the best of friends as boys. We had seen each other often in London when I was a medical student. Then he emigrated to Australia. After that we had little direct contact, but I heard on the family grapevine what he was up to. Surfing, farming, running a hotel from the farmhouse before becoming a DJ . . . I'd lost track by now. And I couldn't keep up with his various marriages and plethora of children either. Certainly, none of it surprised me. Geoff was always destined to be less conventional than me. I was the focused grammar-school boy. Geoff hadn't even taken his eleven plus. Something he saw on a screen in a television-shop window on the way to the exam had so diverted him that he had arrived too late to enter.

I feared his appearance on the Isle of Man might provoke a clash of cultures – the Australian with the alternative life-style meeting the rather correct colonialists. But I had underestimated Maggie and Austin and forgotten Geoff's easy charm. Within a few hours it was as though they had known each other for years and, as for me – well, we were boys again, joking and laughing together. Geoff played cricket on the beach, told wildly improbable tales of Australian life, mended farm fences, ushered Maggie from the kitchen, insisting on cooking the meal that night, and enthralled both children and dogs.

During those three days Geoff and I took a few long walks together, talking about our family and the past. He told me he'd spent time in the Outback. He had great respect for the culture of the First People and had subsequently met various healers who eschewed Western medicine but achieved remarkable outcomes for the very sick. Geoff loved remarkable outcomes. I remembered how, as boys, we had tried some hair oil, obtained by him, of course. It was supposed to make our hair grow at twice the normal rate, long hair in that era being highly desirable to the young and delightfully irritating to the old. It didn't seem to work for me but Geoff had reported that his had gained inches in a week, *and* it was blonder.

We stopped by a rock on the coast path now, high above the sea, so high we could not even hear it crashing below us, and Geoff told me he had lumps in his neck and his healer friend was going to deal with them as soon as he got back to Australia.

I asked if he wanted me to look at them.

He shrugged and pulled down his sweater, guiding my fingers towards his neck.

'Hope this didn't start with that hair oil,' I said. But Geoff did not laugh. 'That stuff was amazing. I wish I'd kept some!'

My fingers had landed now, just below the angle of his jaw. I could easily feel the lumps. They were firm and rubbery.

'Does that hurt?' I asked.

'Nah.'

'Do you have them anywhere else?'

Geoff, being Geoff, began to take off his clothes. He held up his arms and guided my fingers to his hairy armpit. Nodules. Firm and rubbery.

'Got them here, too –'

He prepared to take off his trousers, but I stopped him.

'I don't need to see any more . . . I assume they're in your groin?'

'Yeah. My healer says that I need to take some silver

because it'll bring me closer to the earth. He reckons these lumps are a sign that I've been thinking too much lately about the past and I need to get grounded in the present . . .'

He was putting on his clothes again, his lean, brown body silhouetted against the clouds behind him. Beneath us, the water was a deep, deep blue. There is a local name for the light sea mist that covers the Isle of Man. It is called Manannan's Cloak. Now, something like Manannan's Cloak was inside my head: you couldn't really see it but you could certainly feel it. Sadness. And its cruel twin, loss.

My cousin and oldest friend was looking at me hard now. 'Dick . . . ?'

'This . . . healer. He's not a doctor?'

'No way, he doesn't believe in that stuff.'

'But he's steeped in Aboriginal medicine?'

'Hell, no! He spent some time studying with the First People but he takes full credit for evolving his theories himself. He went into the Outback alone to think and he came back with . . . so much understanding. So much knowledge. I wish you could meet him, Dick.'

I was secretly glad I would not meet the healer who believed that nostalgic thinking had caused those lumps and now claimed silver would cure them.

'Geoff, do you ever go to a normal doctor?'

'Nah.'

'Will you do me a favour? Just this once? Will you go when you get back?'

He argued, saying that he fully trusted his healer, but I persuaded him to go for my sake and he finally agreed.

I was sufficiently concerned to contact him soon after his return to Australia.

'Well, you know what doctors are like, Dick, you probably

do it yourself. Find a bunch of long words to describe something perfectly simple.'

The long words were 'diffuse large B-cell lymphoma'. The
perfectly simple something was cancer. I had been fairly sure
he had a lymphoma, or maybe it was leukaemia, but both
were eminently treatable. So I felt confident the cancer could
be either cured or kept at bay for a long, long time. If he
stopped listening to his healer.

'Yeah, the doc said it's a slow one, so I figure I've got time
for Brian to deal with it.'

'Brian?'

'My spiritual and physical healer.'

Brian seemed a colourless name for a healer.

'So, this Brian, he wants to give you silver?'

'Yeah, he's started the treatment and he's very confident
it's working. In fact, I think the lumps have already gone
down a bit.'

'Geoff, it's only a slow cancer if it's treated. If it's not,
then –'

'I'm treating it, man, I'm treating it with silver. Brian knows
what he's doing.'

Geoff lived for less than a year. I was glad that we'd seen
each other on the Isle of Man, I was just sorry that it turned
out to be for the last time. His death was unnecessarily early
and I felt great anger at this Brian, with his silver and his
nonsense. Especially when Geoff's widow, whom I phoned
to express my condolences and talk about him, told me that
they had sold the farm to pay for his treatment.

'Didn't he try conventional medicine at all?' I asked crustily.

'Oh yes. We were made to at the end but, needless to say,
it was useless,' she said.

'Because you were too late!'

27

But she wasn't listening.

'Brian warned us we were wasting our time with doctors, and as usual he was right. And, you know, when Geoff was dying and Brian came in and found they'd put him on oxygen, he said: "I'm switching that stuff off, they're poisoning him."'

There was nothing more I could say. Calling Brian a charlatan at this stage would be counterproductive. I'd phoned Geoff a few times while he was receiving his 'treatment' and it had been clear to me then that he had invested so much, psychologically and philosophically, in his healer that he could not now give up his faith. Like an addicted gambler, all he could do was invest more and more.

Geoff sacrificed his life to his beliefs. These were not based on any solid evidence and they were not moral or political: they were simply personal, so much a part of the man that they could not be relinquished. And when, soon after Geoff's death, I was contacted once more about Fergusson Bell, I realized that the same had been true of Mr Bell – although here a helpless son was required to sacrifice his life for his father's philosophy. So perhaps I was feeling a bit less sympathetic towards the Bell family when I was phoned by one of the experts in metabolism who had examined Fergusson's case.

The Bells now had a new son, and there was no slipping under the NHS radar this time. The specialist thought it essential to test the second baby for Fergusson's problem: both parents must have carried this recessive gene and the chances were therefore 75 per cent that the child would either inherit the full disorder or be a carrier. The truth about Fergusson's new brother could rapidly be ascertained by a fructose intolerance test.

But the test required contact with hospitals and doctors – as well as an IV. The father flatly refused to allow this intrusion by conventional medicine and was fighting hard against it. One way to safeguard the child and accommodate his father's objections was to establish whether Fergusson and his brother shared the same fructose intolerance by sequencing both babies' DNA. This was then a massive task, but a laboratory generously offered to try. The specialist now asked: had I kept a tissue sample from the late Fergusson which they could work from? It would enable them to isolate the intolerant gene.

I had indeed, and the second son proved to be a carrier. That meant he could one day pass the trait to his children and, if they were unlucky enough to have a mother with the same trait, they would be fructose intolerant. However, the boy himself was unaffected by it.

A benign ending to a sad story, then, which is only slightly marred by the father's subsequent adventures in alternative medicine. Many people have a healthy disrespect for conventional medicine, which they sometimes temper when they are ill and need treatment. Mr Bell's public scorn for the mainstream was not modified after the death of his son. My sympathy for this bereaved parent entirely evaporated when I learned that, without any of the qualifications this implies, he had changed his title from Mr to Dr and asserted publicly – and probably still does so – that his methods can cure the cancerous and very sick. He encourages those who share his view to turn their backs on chemotherapy, radiotherapy or any other recognized cancer treatment and to adopt his dietary treatment instead. At least those he treats presumably have a choice. My cousin Geoff had a choice too, and he chose to die. Mr Bell's baby son, of course, had no choice. And that is the crux of the Fergusson Bell case: the right of the Bells to reject conventional medicine had bumped up against Fergusson's right to survive. It is a choice every parent faces, in a less direct way, when deciding whether to vaccinate a child. I believe that those who have full information, as opposed to misinformation, must surely decide that the risks of, for instance, death or serious complication from measles, both to one's own child and to society in general, greatly outweigh the risks of vaccination. Yet many parents choose not to vaccinate.

How hard it is to give up our beliefs. How hard it must have been for the self-styled doctor Mr Bell to admit his son had a problem conventional medicine could deal with and his own system could not. Admitting this would not just have involved shaking his faith, it would have required him to reassess it. And he was not prepared to make such a fundamental change in his thinking. Perhaps, without his beliefs, he would have wondered who he really was. We define and redefine ourselves throughout our lives: sometimes, when we eventually reach old age, our memory is lost and with it that definition. And then who are we?

It was Geoff's death that made me think long and hard again about the Bell case and, perhaps, to change my mind. I now find myself half wishing that the detective inspector had been successful in her prosecution attempt.

2

Fergusson's unnecessary death illustrates not just how complex and prone to error are pre-conception and pregnancy, but how, once born, the quality of care we give babies is, as well as their greatest security, the greatest threat to their well-being. Sometimes love is just as dangerous as fury because babies' dependency means they are prey to the inexperience, idiosyncrasies, idiocies or weaknesses of even the most well-meaning caregivers. I've lost count of such cases, the ones which fall somewhere in between great bad luck and a carelessness so extreme that it might be called wilful neglect.

The baby who was put on the top bunk bed and slipped down between the wall and the mattress, asphyxiating herself. The baby who died of burns when she fell behind the radiator. The infant who was strangled by the cord from the nightlight hanging over his cot. The baby in the arms of a drunken father who fell downstairs. The toddler who was left alone with his lunchbox around his neck and strangled himself. The baby who was dropped on to hard, metal loudspeakers when her mother tripped over the family dog. The baby who drowned in the bath when her parent went to answer the phone. The baby who succumbed to dehydration and starvation in a flat alone with a father who had died of a drugs overdose. The list is endless and hideously varied. No one intended any of those small children to die. But effectively, most of them died from, in differing degrees, lack of care.

And what about the babies who die because that really is

someone's intention? The baby has arrived healthy in this world by a series of miracles and now no one wants them to be here. Those who torture or kill babies seldom see them as dependent scraps of humanity. A few quite simply relish the thought of inflicting pain. A wife who hid under the bed-clothes so she could not hear her baby's cries as her husband hurt their daughter explained to a court: 'I told him he was a sadist. He admitted he enjoyed giving people pain . . . and he said the baby used to annoy him and aggravate him.'

But those who receive pleasure from inflicting pain are the minority of baby-killers. Having read numerous interviews with many such bereaved parents, I would say that most often the child's constant crying and demands are interpreted by the carer who kills not as expressions of need but as calculated, deliberate and malicious acts designed to provoke.

Oddly, there is sometimes another child in the family, an older sibling, who escapes fury because the carer believes that only this particular baby has the evil intent of upsetting them. And for some parents, a baby's cries symbolize much more than the child's own helplessness. Perhaps the expression of need reminds the parent of their own unmet needs. Perhaps the baby's uncompromising demands recall for the parent an unbearable host of uncompromising demands faced daily from others. Perhaps there is no other scapegoat on whom a parent can safely vent uncontainable anger. Perhaps the baby's cries penetrate the weakness of the family's structure and relationships. A new baby is a symbol of hope, but the reality of a baby's demands can be isolating, stripping all joy from the parent. Yes, we have all been driven near the end of our tether by persistent crying and this is certainly exacerbated in situations of poverty and extreme stress. But isolation can have the same effect on anyone, even in opulent surroundings. However, there can be no excuse for infanticide. So let us hear what those who admit to this crime tell us.

I examined a four-week-old baby girl who had died of a fractured skull and a subdural haemorrhage, clearly the result of a hard blow. I noted bruises to her head, face and neck which I recognized as gripping injuries. She also had many rib fractures: I estimated these were ten days old. It was clear that this child had been persistently hurt and then killed.

The couple had one girl already who was just over a year old and who appeared unharmed. Things had changed recently in the family when the father, Aaron, lost his job in a bank. The couple's early interviews demonstrate their denial, certainly to the police but perhaps also to themselves. Here is what the father said when first asked to explain his daughter's facial bruises.

FATHER:	Well, the only thing we could think of that could cause it was maybe the way we hold her when we wind her . . . the marks would go for a couple of days and then they'd come back. But we couldn't fathom out what it was, it just seemed strange that she was getting them near enough in the same place, but we couldn't fathom it out because we didn't wind her like that any more . . .
INTERVIEWER:	So you can't account for how she got the bruises on her cheeks?
FATHER:	No, I just can't understand it . . . !
INTERVIEWER:	Now, at the post-mortem, the pathologist found she had some broken ribs.

FATHER:	Oh, really?
INTERVIEWER:	Can you account for these?
FATHER:	No, I didn't know, I don't know how she could get them either, really.
INTERVIEWER:	. . . There were six broken ribs . . .
FATHER:	Bloody hell!
INTERVIEWER:	Six broken ribs on one side at the front, four on the other side and eight at the back on one side and three the other.
FATHER:	Jesus Christ!
INTERVIEWER:	And she certainly didn't do it herself.
FATHER:	No, well, I mean, we used to wind her, but you don't, we didn't sort of hit her, it was just stroking her back . . . she did cry in her sleep but we just thought it was like . . . nightmares. No, I honestly don't know how that happened.
INTERVIEWER:	Well, I think you do.
FATHER:	No, why would I lie?
INTERVIEWER:	It's not easy being a dad with a newborn, but if things have got on top of you, we ask you to have the courage to tell us.
FATHER:	No, I mean, if I was upset or anything, I certainly wouldn't take it out on the kids . . .
INTERVIEWER:	The post-mortem has also shown a fractured skull.
FATHER:	How . . . how the bloody hell did she get that?

INTERVIEWER:	That's what we're asking you.
FATHER:	It's [*sic*] my daughter, I loved her . . . I don't see any point covering up or lying if I've done something wrong.

No confessions there. So what about the mother? She was asked to explain why she had failed to take the baby to clinic appointments.

MOTHER:	I said to Aaron that, you know, going to the clinic with those bruises, I said, look at her, it looks as though we've battered her, you know, hurt her.
INTERVIEWER:	You said that?
MOTHER:	Yes, I did, but it was only . . . I didn't want people to think that we had hurt her, because we hadn't.
INTERVIEWER:	You must have thought that you had, or somebody else had.
MOTHER:	I knew I hadn't and I have no proof that Aaron had, I hadn't seen any, you know, violence.
INTERVIEWER:	But did you think that Aaron had battered the baby?
MOTHER:	No, not battered her. I thought that perhaps he'd started winding her that way again and the bruises had come back . . .
INTERVIEWER:	But you told us you asked him how he was winding her and he explained, so you can't really have thought that.

SOLICITOR:	With respect, my client is only telling you what she thought.
MOTHER:	I suppose in a tiny part of my mind I thought: had he done it? But you try to blank it out, I suppose.
INTERVIEWER:	Is that what you did? Tried to blank it out?
MOTHER:	Because I hadn't seen him, I hadn't heard her . . . and he's so good with them. It may have crossed my mind once, but that was all.

That evening, the father was interviewed again. He adopted the same astonished tone when asked about his daughter's injuries. The interview ended abruptly. The next morning, he was interviewed once more.

INTERVIEWER:	Last night, Aaron, you asked us to finish your interview.
FATHER:	I needed time to think.
INTERVIEWER:	And you also wanted to talk to your solicitor, I believe. Now you've had time to think, is there anything you want to tell us?
FATHER:	Well, just that it was me that injured the baby but . . . I know this is going to sound terrible, but I didn't know what I was doing sort of thing. It's not an excuse. I'm not excusing myself, but I seem to get sort of panicky and I was a bit depressed because I'd lost my job and sometimes it got

too much for me and I just lashed out. But I don't remember the details of it and ... all I felt afterwards was remorse. I can't explain it. I just sort of snapped.

INTERVIEWER: The baby cried a lot, did she?

FATHER: When she started crying it used to really annoy me or upset me and I think I have gone ... like I say ... I've flipped and just lashed out. I don't remember how or why. Afterwards all I remember is just feeling sorry about it.

INTERVIEWER: The baby's ribs were broken about ten days ago. Can you tell us how that happened?

FATHER: I don't really know. To be honest, it could be any time. I didn't really know what I was doing ...

INTERVIEWER: How do you think the broken ribs were caused?

FATHER: I might have slapped her or cuddled her too hard or crushed her, well, not crushed her but squeezed her to shut her up. I never actually meant to hurt her.

INTERVIEWER: But a baby that age –

FATHER: I loved her.

INTERVIEWER: I need to know exactly how she got those injuries, Aaron. Can you help me?

FATHER: I might have hit her.

INTERVIEWER:	Did you hit her?
FATHER:	I know I must have hit her. I'm owning up to it but I can't remember when and I can't remember why.
INTERVIEWER:	It's the how . . . ?
FATHER:	It's not something I'd do knowingly, you know, I wouldn't just say, oh well, I've got to shut her up so I'll hit her. I wouldn't do that, I'm not that sort of person. So something happened to me that made me flip . . . I know I was going a bit funny with everything on top of me, worrying and losing my job, but I don't remember doing it.
INTERVIEWER:	But each time you hurt her, you felt guilty afterwards?
FATHER:	Then I'd just try to calm her down and console her. I don't remember doing it, just the guilt afterwards.
INTERVIEWER:	But first you bruised her face, then you broke her ribs and then you broke her skull . . . and you don't remember?
FATHER:	I'd never, never have done anything to hurt her, believe me. If I knew what I was doing. But I obviously didn't.
INTERVIEWER:	You told your friend that you hated the baby.
FATHER:	No, that's not true.
INTERVIEWER:	You didn't hate her?
FATHER:	When she was crying, I didn't hate it [sic] but I resented her for crying.

38

INTERVIEWER: Your friend said you used the word
                 'hated'.

FATHER: I might have done, yeah.

The surviving daughter was immediately removed from this couple's care and, after a very difficult court case – difficult because neither parent admitted in court to any knowledge of the baby's injuries – the father was convicted of murder and child cruelty, the mother of child cruelty.

The interviews show that the father knew very well how he should behave: as an adult who loved his children. And he also knew how he did behave: violently. It is his management of this strange gap between who he wanted to be and who he was which must have enabled him to continue hurting the child time and time again. Perhaps it's a gap which all parents are familiar with: Aaron is an extreme case and the consequences were tragic.

Here is another case. Sarah was a young mother whose daughter died at four months. The dissonance she displayed in her interviews was similar to Aaron's, but she played things very differently from him.

Her own mother gave Sarah's history to the police, explaining that she had shown disturbed behaviour at primary school and had been diagnosed then with learning difficulties. At secondary school she was badly bullied and by the age of fourteen had become highly sexually active. In fact, two pregnancies had already been terminated before, at the age of seventeen, during a brief relationship, she became pregnant with Katie. She lived alone in a council flat with the baby. She had a visiting boyfriend and a supportive family quite nearby.

When I examined Katie's body, the baby's heart histology

39

did show a significant lymphocytic infiltrate. I strongly suspected viral myocarditis. I wrote in the first draft of my post-mortem report: 'Viral infections of the heart may be fatal but many individuals recover from such infections and they may, in many, have no obvious clinical effect. Viral myocarditis therefore can be fatal but is not necessarily so.'

The virus might have meant Katie's murder went undetected or anyway unproven. However, the mother, Sarah, went to the police station with her own mother the next morning and confessed to killing Katie. She was immediately arrested.

INTERVIEWER: And what made you come to the police station, Sarah?

SARAH: Guilt.

INTERVIEWER: In what way?

SARAH: That I did it.

INTERVIEWER: I know this is hard for you. Would you like to tell me what happened? From yesterday morning?

SARAH: Katie wasn't taking her solids all day and she was very whingey because she was crying most of the time. And I just got really stressed so in the end I put her in the bedroom and left her to cry . . .

INTERVIEWER: Where were you?

SARAH: In the lounge. Having a cigarette and thinking and thinking. I was getting so worked up.

INTERVIEWER: What did you do?

SARAH:	I went in the bedroom because I was really stressed out and I just wanted to shut her up and I took her out of her cot and laid her on the bed and I got the sheet that I wrap her up in and I put it over her face.
INTERVIEWER:	Will you show me what you did with your hands?
SARAH:	(*demonstrates*) I put my right hand on her nose and my thumb under her mouth so she couldn't breathe.
INTERVIEWER:	And what did Katie do?
SARAH:	Nothing.
INTERVIEWER:	Did she struggle?
SARAH:	Yeah, she kicked her legs.
INTERVIEWER:	How long did you keep your hands in this position?
SARAH:	A few seconds. I didn't think I kept them there that long to have killed her.
INTERVIEWER:	What were you thinking when you did that?
SARAH:	I was just so stressed, I wasn't thinking of anything.
INTERVIEWER:	What happened then?
SARAH:	Well, after she stopped kicking I took the sheet away and I saw that she had her mouth open and I shut it and it made me have a flashback of what happened a couple of weeks ago, so I tried to resuscitate her but she just wouldn't breathe.

INTERVIEWER:	What happened a couple of weeks ago?
SARAH:	I was sitting watching TV and I had this feeling something was wrong. I don't normally keep checking on Katie, but something told me to this time. I'd put her on her front because she likes sleeping that way and, when I went in to check on her, I saw her right hand was blue. So I picked her up and she was cold. And I shook her, but she was just so floppy, like there was no life in her at all.
INTERVIEWER:	What did you do?
SARAH:	I rushed to phone my mum and she told me to phone an ambulance. So I did and they told me what to do. I had to resuscitate her, and I did, I succeeded.
INTERVIEWER:	I see.
SARAH:	But unfortunately, yesterday, I didn't.
INTERVIEWER:	Was anyone else there?
SARAH:	No, but I knew Mike was coming round at about eight o'clock so I made up a plan. I know it sounds horrible but I was so scared that I just put her back in the cot and then I thought that I'd hint for Mike to go and see her so that he could find her and he wouldn't suspect it was me.
INTERVIEWER:	And is that what happened?

SARAH:	He came in and I said: 'Do you want to see Katie?' And he said: 'Yeah. Is she asleep?' I said: 'I don't know. Turn the light on if you want.' Then I was tidying up and Mike was in there and he said: 'She looks a bit funny.' And I said: 'That's just the way she sleeps.' He picked her up and sat her on his lap and he said: 'Sarah, she doesn't look right to me.' So I went and pretended that it shocked me and I had a cup of tea and I dropped it on the floor so he wouldn't suspect me. Then I grabbed her off him and I tried to resuscitate her.
INTERVIEWER:	How long after she died was it before Mike came in?
SARAH:	Just five, ten minutes. She was still warm, so I thought she was still alive.
INTERVIEWER:	I see.
SARAH:	I did everything to get her back.
INTERVIEWER:	You wanted her back, then?
SARAH:	I did. I don't know why I did it.
INTERVIEWER:	Is everything you've told me the truth?
SARAH:	I'm afraid it is. I feel better for saying it. And awful.
INTERVIEWER:	Do you have anything else to say?
SARAH:	I just want to tell you that I didn't mean to do it. She meant everything to me. I didn't mean to kill her, I didn't

	know I did it for that long. It only felt like a few seconds. I loved her very much and I miss her and when I saw her today I just wanted her to open her eyes and cry.
INTERVIEWER:	You said you did it with your hands . . . so why did you use the sheet?
SARAH:	Because I didn't want to see her face.

Once I was told of Sarah's confession, I immediately re-examined the body. There were no petechial haemorrhages – these are red dots which can be found anywhere but, if on the eyes or face in particular, may indicate asphyxiation; however, they are seldom found on babies. There was no evidence of injury to the lips, gums or nose. Nothing, in fact, pointed to the possibility that Katie had been smothered. The mother's story could not be verified. I wrote:

> Sarah said that it 'only felt like a few seconds': in my opinion, it is most unlikely that death in these circumstances would occur in a few seconds.
>
> In this case there are two possible causes of death. Viral myocarditis is of natural origin. Smothering or suffocation is not. A third possibility is that Katie was more susceptible to asphyxia due to her viral myocarditis. I am unable, on the evidence I have, to determine which of these possibilities is correct and I am unable therefore to give a precise cause of death. I give:
>
> **1a. Not Determined.**

A specialist forensic paediatric pathologist was consulted. He confirmed the presence of the virus, which he agreed could occasionally be fatal. He then considered the mother's story and wrote:

> Suffocation or smothering may leave no positive pathological evidence in a young infant, in particular if some soft material is used to occlude the mouth and nose and if the force applied is not excessive. In that context, the possibility that Katie died as a result of asphyxiation cannot be excluded. I agree with Dr Shepherd that the pathological findings alone cannot assist any further in determining the true cause of death in this case.

When, in another interview, Sarah was asked again what she had been thinking when she decided to smother the child, she described how she sat in the next room as Katie cried, smoking and trying to calm down. 'I was thinking, oh my God, shut up, shut up, stop doing this to me. I don't want it. I want a peaceful life. I want my life too!'

This is something many murderers of babies have in common, this presentation of themselves as a victim of the child's manipulations. Can they be right that a baby actually has an evil motive? I do not believe so but, once that baby becomes a moving, enquiring, thinking infant, when does criminality begin?

In most of the UK, criminality is recognized from ten years and upwards and in Scotland the age has recently been raised to twelve. However, in the following case, I was forced to acknowledge, extremely reluctantly, that it may be possible for a three-year-old to commit murder. Of course, there are three-year-olds who accidentally kill a sibling when helpfully teaching baby to swim in the bath or trying to clean baby in the washing machine, but that is not murder. Murder is a crime which requires not just the death of the victim but intent to kill on the part of the perpetrator.

I travelled to Devon to carry out a post-mortem on a five-month-old baby who had died in a seaside village. I found him to be rather small for his age, because he had been born prematurely, but otherwise to have no illness or injury. Except for his head. Which had been quite shockingly damaged. One side of his skull had multiple fractures, and inside that his brain showed extensive contusion and laceration as well as a number of haemorrhages. The other side of his face was extensively bruised and his upper lip was torn.

My initial response was that the bruises were caused by gripping; I suggested that a large, adult hand had seized the baby's face. The more terrible injuries were consistent with blunt trauma, a trauma that had been administered with con-siderable force.

The police then showed me an interview with the alleged perpetrator. They explained that he was just three years old. I felt it was scarcely possible that a toddler could have com-mitted a crime of such magnitude, nor demonstrated the force required. The police then told me the circumstances. The death had occurred at the village playgroup. Mothers were on a rota to help and the mother of this baby, who had an older child in the playgroup, had wheeled him in his buggy, asleep, into a side room, closed the door and then rolled up her sleeves and got to work with crayons and powder paint.

The baby was in a sort of office with a hard concrete floor. There were filing cabinets and cupboards for equipment storage. There was some dispute as to whether the baby had been strapped into his pushchair and, if he was, whether the strap was effective.

During the session, the mother and supervisor and

various other helpers went in and out of the office to fetch things, without disturbing the baby. Apart from the mother, most had apparently said that they had not even looked at him because they were so busy.

Two hours after the baby was left, the supervisor returned to the office, and this time she could not but look at the baby: he was on the floor and bleeding profusely. She reported that leaning over the baby was three-year-old Jamie. An ambulance very rapidly arrived but the baby could not have survived such injuries and he died soon afterwards.

I was never a party to the details of the police investigation. I have no idea how many people they interviewed or how well they analysed the movements of those who went in and out of the side room. The main witness was Jamie's four-year-old brother, who did not attend the playgroup but said Jamie had told him in secret that he had thrown the baby out of the buggy and cracked his head open.

Both Jamie and his brother were questioned separately by a specialist in interviewing children.

The interviewer first played extensively with Jamie in a room full of toys and gradually used the toys to persuade him to talk about what had happened at playgroup. Finally, she asked the big question. The italic notes are the interviewer's own.

INTERVIEWER: Jamie, how did the baby fall out of the buggy?
JAMIE: The mum went like that and it fell out.

(Jamie was holding a toy ambulance and now he tipped it over.)

JAMIE: The baby is dead.
INTERVIEWER: How do you know the baby is dead?

(Jamie's reply was indistinct. He played with the Play-Doh. I asked Jamie if he had hung up his coat at playschool and said I'd heard he had found a Batman cloak.)

JAMIE:	I had a cloak on.
INTERVIEWER:	Where did you get that from?
JAMIE:	Out the cupboard.
INTERVIEWER:	Which cupboard was that, then?
JAMIE:	My teacher's.
INTERVIEWER:	Is the cupboard in the same room where you play with Play-Doh or is it in another room?
JAMIE:	Another room.
INTERVIEWER:	Was there anyone else in that room?
JAMIE:	Just the baby.
INTERVIEWER:	Did you say hello to the baby?
JAMIE:	And he fell out of his buggy.
INTERVIEWER:	How did the baby fall out of his buggy?
JAMIE:	The mum tipped it over.
INTERVIEWER:	Was there only the mum there or were there other people?
JAMIE:	Other peoples.
INTERVIEWER:	Who were they?
JAMIE:	My teachers.
INTERVIEWER:	Did you see the baby on the floor, Jamie?
JAMIE:	No.
INTERVIEWER:	How do you know he was tipped out of the buggy then?
JAMIE:	The mum tipped it over.

(Jamie was distracted by his toys, then.)

INTERVIEWER:	Did all this happen when you went in to get that Batman cloak?
JAMIE:	Yeah.
INTERVIEWER:	So you went into the room and the baby was there, and it was just you and the baby?
JAMIE:	The teacher pushed him.
INTERVIEWER:	Did you try to pick up the baby?
JAMIE:	No.
INTERVIEWER:	Did you push the buggy over?
JAMIE:	The mum did.
INTERVIEWER:	Did she knock it over? Or did she pick it up?
JAMIE:	Pick it up and then she let it out of her hands.
INTERVIEWER:	Did the baby cry, Jamie?
JAMIE:	He didn't.
INTERVIEWER:	Where did the baby look hurt?
JAMIE:	Near the coats.
INTERVIEWER:	Is that where the baby banged his head?

(There were many indistinct answers now.)

JAMIE:	Blood comed out of him.
INTERVIEWER:	Where was the blood?
JAMIE:	Out of his mouth.
INTERVIEWER:	Did the mummy know you were there? Or couldn't she see you?
JAMIE:	No.
INTERVIEWER:	Where were you?
JAMIE:	Hiding.
INTERVIEWER:	Where?

JAMIE:	Round the corner.
INTERVIEWER:	I'm puzzled, Jamie, I don't know who tipped the buggy over.
JAMIE:	The mummy.
INTERVIEWER:	The mummy, not the teachers?
JAMIE:	One of the teachers came in and looked after the baby.

This is an edited extract from a very long, often contradictory and, I would say, extremely inconclusive interview. Anyone who has tried to get rational sense out of a three-year-old will know how challenging this must have been, even for a trained child interviewer. Nevertheless, Jamie's interview was relayed to the coroner's court, along with his four-year-old brother's nebulous accusations.

The coroner gave an open verdict and the police described the baby's death to local newspapers, who gave the story very little space, as a 'tragic accident involving a three-year-old boy'.

For myself, I could not then and cannot now entirely believe the child was guilty. I have no idea who the other adults were at playgroup, no information about their movements or what motive someone might have had for hurting that baby and I know nothing about the baby's family.

Although at first I was convinced that the force with which the baby was killed could only have come from an adult, particularly given the tell-tale facial bruising that looked so much like gripping injuries, before I had reached the second draft of the report the police had phoned. They asked when they would receive the report and reminded me to include the fact that a child throwing a small baby on to a hard floor could inflict those injuries.

I did admit that possibility. It existed, albeit remotely. I was sure that whoever had killed the baby, they had intended at the very least to hurt him — such injuries could not have been sustained through even energetic play. But, in my heart, I am certainly not convinced that Jamie had the strength required to cause those injuries. And as I reread the notes now, the conclusion I reach is that the first age of criminality is not three years old.

And then the whining school-boy, with his satchel
And shining morning face, creeping like snail
Unwillingly to school:

3

It was a winter night and it seemed I had just gone to bed when the phone rang. A voice asked me to drive to Kent. A child had died in hospital in suspicious circumstances.

I dressed and got in the car without asking any questions. 'Suspicious circumstances' is a phrase which generates a sense of hurry, although the dead are always patient. As I drove south, I half assumed that there would be a baby in the mortuary. Since the death had occurred in hospital, I expected that some unfortunate parents had discovered late in the evening that their baby was not breathing, called an ambulance, and all attempts at resuscitation had failed. Although Sudden Infant Death Syndrome is a natural enough occurrence, at that time it was always regarded as suspicious.

A line of tired and ashen police faces was awaiting me. We sat in the bereavement room and an assistant handed me a mug of hot tea as the detective explained that in fact the deceased was a seven-year-old girl. She had been reported missing in the early evening and a search had ensued. Finally, at nine thirty that evening, she had been found by a police dog in a park. The dog's handler immediately called the paramedics, who arrived with blue flashing lights and a lot of kit. The child was whisked to hospital, where all attempts at resuscitation failed. The inspector told me that the paramedics, in retrospect, believed that she had almost certainly been dead for some time when she was found.

If she was beyond resuscitation, I couldn't help wishing

that they had left her *in situ*. There had not even been any pictures taken of the scene.

A detective showed me a diagram indicating the position of the body, drawn helpfully by the police dog handler who had found her. Although it was so bad that I wondered if perhaps the dog had drawn it.

'What's this?' I asked, staring at what seemed to be a jagged row of teeth, apparently hovering over a small stick insect, which I took to be the body of the child.

'Well, that's a broken branch. See, it had broken off and fallen quite near where she was found.'

'Ah. And . . . I can't tell from this . . . was she on the path? Or in the bushes?'

A detective sergeant had been quick enough to beat the ambulance to the scene.

'In the bushes, Doc. Definitely in the bushes.'

'And this seems to be the most enormous Coke can in the world . . . ?' The dog handler had lacked any skills in drawing perspective.

'Yeah, crushed, she was lying on it. Probably just a bit of litter. Anyway, Forensics have taken it.'

'So was she actually under the fallen branch?'

'Yeah, sort of.'

'You don't think it fell on her?'

'No, nothing like that, it's been down a while. It looked as if she might have crawled underneath it, though.'

'She was hiding?'

'Her mum reported her missing at about half past five and said she'd done it before.'

'Done what?'

'Run away from home. She had a little bag packed, see, he's drawn it right beside her here.'

He pointed to an odd shape, like a small treasure chest.

'How far from home did she get?'

'About two minutes.'

I smiled. My daughter had once threatened to run away, but this had taken her as far as the garden shed.

'So she was lying under bushes, as if she'd been crawling under the fallen tree branch, and her bag was beside her?'

'Yeah.'

'But . . . she was flat on her back?'

'Yeah.'

That didn't sound right to me. I could see the detectives were tired. They weren't sure if someone had killed Clare Romeril or an accident had befallen her. As we met up in the post-mortem room, I thought they were probably all hoping it had been an accident. Then they could go home to bed, instead of launching a murder inquiry. I knew that, statistically, they were likely to be right. The figures tell us that the most common cause of the unnatural death of a seven-year-old girl is certainly an accident.

I found Clare Romeril's upper body still covered in ECG tabs, resuscitation marks and the evidence of intravenous injections. I took her temperature. She had been declared dead in the hospital at 10 p.m. but it was clear that she must have died some hours before that.

'How many hours?' asked the detective sergeant keenly. I sighed. This is always the most pressing question for the police and the most hated for the forensic pathologist. It is difficult and often impossible to estimate the time of death. The police can't understand why we can't just give a straight answer to such a straight question. Useless to explain that there is a vortex of variables to contend with.

However, allowing for the fact that Clare was a child and

therefore her body cooled faster, recognizing that she was well covered if not actually fat, acknowledging that the evening had not been cold for winter but noting that she had worn only pink trainers, underpants, a My Little Pony T-shirt and a pink skirt, taking into account the wind that had blown last night, the drop in temperature when it had rained a few times . . . after considering all that and then consulting the hideously complex diagram pathologists use for this purpose, which bears a similarity in both appearance and accuracy to an astrological chart, I finally estimated her time of death at between 5 and 7 p.m.

'Hmmmm,' said the detective sergeant. 'She was only reported missing at five thirty.'

He exchanged pained looks with the detective inspector and I realized they were sceptical. They had as little faith in the diagram as I did.

I set about examining the exterior of Clare's body. There was nothing about her appearance to suggest she was anything other than well fed and well cared for. I could tell everyone was hoping that she had not been sexually assaulted. She had not. I swabbed, of course, to be sure, but there was no sign of bruising or injury of any kind to vagina or anus, and I said so. The room gave a collective sigh of relief. If Clare had been murdered, sexual assault would have been the likely motive. Without it, everyone's belief was reinforced that her death must have been accidental. Let your child out of your sight, we agreed, and they get themselves into trouble.

I slipped off her necklace, which consisted of little more than a tiny blue stone on a piece of cord, the sort of thing any little girl might wear. The stone left a deep imprint on her throat. Then, if it wasn't already, it became clear to all that the necklace was responsible for her death. Beneath it was a clear, deep, abraded mark. The tell-tale line dipped between the bottom of one ear and the bottom of the other and, like the necklace, it was three millimetres wide.

So, Clare's necklace had somehow strangled her. Now I'd found the obvious cause of death, it would have been nice to pack up and go home, but there is so much more to a post-mortem. I have to see what else the body can tell us and I have to establish that there is no natural disease which might have contributed to death. All the organs must be examined, every bruise or mark, on the inside of the body as well as the outside. It was going to be a long night.

As I worked, the detectives speculated that Clare might have strangled herself when she crawled under the bushes, snagging her necklace beneath the broken branch with its myriad small, spiky offshoots.

'It's very easy to do that,' I agreed and, without looking up, I sensed that the detectives were nodding. They were sure now. Clare's death was accidental. I pointed out the classic signs of asphyxiation on her face and eyes, those small red dots we call petechial haemorrhages.

Ligature strangulation, then, was scarcely in doubt. The question was: had anyone else been involved? And the only way to determine that as a pathologist was to look for any signs of violence: a scuffle or attempted self-defence.

There was an insignificant bruise on Clare's left upper arm and signs of an old graze on her face. There were some old, healing bruises on her lower legs: nothing uncommon in an energetic child, and Clare was probably energetic: she had been labelled 'difficult' and her mother had said that she regularly ran away. I didn't stop then to wonder why this might be.

'Oh my God, look at that, someone's given her a good

hiding after all!' said one of the detectives as I turned her small body over to study her back. It's true that there was a blue smudge the size of your hand near the midline.

'That's one helluva bruise,' the coroner's officer agreed.

But it wasn't. It was a blue nevus, something we often see in the bodies of children in particular. The position gave it away; the midline of the back, especially the lower back, is a common site for a nevus. It often looks like an irregular round blue mole, but sometimes it simply presents as a patch of skin discoloration and in these cases it is frequently confused with bruising, even by experienced pathologists.

'That's actually a sort of mole,' I said. 'Sometimes it's called a blue nevus. Or a Mongolian blue spot.'

'Sounds like it belongs in the farmyard, some sort of hen,' the coroner's officer said. The detectives did not reply. They were looking at me disbelievingly.

'It's just the pigment's deeper so it looks blue,' I added.

'Looks a lot like a bruise to me,' said the detective sergeant after a pause.

'Really, it's not,' I assured them. I knew I was right. But the mood in the room changed, just a little. I glanced at the detective inspector and saw from his face that he had begun to doubt me. He was alert now for any other bruises or signs of violence for fear I might downplay these. I tried not to bristle under his suspicion.

All Clare's organs were normal: they were the usual size and had the health of youth. A solid, red liver bearing none of the scars of misuse, a firm little heart which should have been beating, and arteries and veins through which the blood had flowed freely without blockage, bulges or the crackling stiffness which occurs later in life. Her skin had a child's purity, unmarked by the sun, mishaps or alcohol.

There was no sign of injury to the scalp, no fracture of the skull, and the brain lay safely cradled inside it. By the age of seven this organ has lost the soft, gelatinous feel of a baby's. It is of course bigger, although brains don't grow as much over a lifetime as the rest of the body: they are 25 per cent of adult weight at birth, which is why a baby's head always seems disproportionately large. By the age of two, the brain is 75 per cent of its adult weight. The brain of a seven-year-old like Clare is close to adult size.

One of the reasons for the brain's expansion is the increase in myelin. Nerve cells transmit instructions to, from and inside the brain and myelin is the fatty substance which over time wraps itself around these cells' long, thin fibres, in just the same way as you might wrap a bottle of wine at Christmas. Suppose you kept wrapping the same bottle over twenty-five years (and never giving it to anyone or drinking it!), you might end up with a hundred layers. Over the first twenty-five years of life that is what the myelin-wrapping cells, called Schwann cells, can achieve. They are mysterious cells and perhaps we do not even yet understand their many functions, but one is certainly to help conduct the electrical messages which rush as fast as 200 mph along the nerve fibres. These fibres run down the spinal column, where they link to the rest of the body. From here, some are very long. For instance, once the instruction to move a finger has reached the spinal column, then just one fibre, which may be more than a metre in length, will relay this to the finger itself. In the same bundle of nerve cells, or neurones, fibres will be working in both directions: sensor neurones will tell the brain that a finger is burning and motor neurones will instruct it to move away from the fire.

All the Schwann cells may not be in place until we reach

the age of twenty-five, but they are already doing a good wrapping job by the age of seven, ensuring messages are arriving at their destination with some reliability via the nerve fibres. One of which was extremely important for Clare Romeril. It was now my job to uncover it.

I cut carefully around the ligature mark and then peeled back the skin. I had to look inside the neck for bruising of the muscles there and, sure enough, I found the tell-tale streaks, red and bloody. Now I had to go deeper and see what further damage there might be.

When a patient is alive, any surgeon operating in this area must have a steady hand. The throat is full of small muscles, and one tiny mistake can dramatically affect the patient's speech or swallowing. To reach that depth I had to remove the huge muscle which blocked my way, which runs from the base of the neck to the ear and stands out so prominently when someone rotates their head. Even in a child it is five centimetres across. I cut it near its base and then used the blunt side of my scalpel to release it from its spiderweb.

The body is full of these webs: organs, muscles, nerves, blood vessels – practically everything inside us is held loosely in place by a fine, intricate weave of connective tissue which has both the appearance and the frailty of something spun by a small and conscientious spider. As soft as cotton wool, it won't anchor anything in a car accident, but in a life without physical trauma it will gently, and with a certain amount of elasticity, persuade vessels, nerves and organs to stay where they should. It is so easy to release a muscle by running your scalpel, or even just a finger, through this tissue plane. Surgeons have to do this on live patients, of course, and, perhaps many years later, if I see those same patients in death, I find

62

that, without the spider's web, vessels and organs have sometimes stuck together and become fixed.

Once I had released it from this soft bed, the big sternomastoid muscle could be moved gently to one side. I was cutting my way deep into the throat now, towards one of the body's greatest holy trinities: the carotid artery, the jugular vein and the vagus nerve.

A vein, artery and nerve snuggling together are known as a neurovascular bundle and this one is joined together inside a very loose structure known as the carotid sheath. A misleading title, sheath. It is reminiscent of strong, leathery knife holsters – when in fact these three vessels are wrapped together in nothing more substantial than tissue paper.

Inside the tissue, the jugular vein looks like a big bruiser, the carotid artery his elegant but rather tubby damsel in white, and, half hidden between them, slender to the point of near-insignificance, is the faithful servant they cannot manage without, the vagus nerve.

Although the human body isn't exactly colour-coded (or I suppose surgery would be so easy that we could all do it), biology books are right to show arteries in red and veins in blue. The jugular vein may be large, at about nine millimetres in diameter, but it is only thinly contained within one-millimetre walls. So, without cutting it, now I felt as though I were flying above it and looking at its contents through light cloud. And what I was seeing was inky blue/black blood. Everyone knows that veins carry deoxygenated blood: this is blue blood. In death it is particularly blue, because the faltering body will have taken every last vestige of oxygen.

The carotid artery carries red, oxygenated blood, but this time you have to open the vessel's white walls to see it.

Arteries have to withstand much higher pressure than veins as blood is pumped around the body by the tireless heart. Result: artery walls are both thick and elastic and the whole vessel has a certain flexibility. In fact, the carotid artery reminds me of my doomed attempts at home winemaking: those white plastic hoses I used were quite flexible when I washed them in hot water. The colour of the blood may be hidden inside the rubbery walls but if the patient is alive you can see the artery expanding and contracting in time to the rhythm of life itself – the beating of the heart.

Now, of course, all was still for Clare. I dissected the artery up its length, always looking for damage, particularly to the very sensitive intima at its centre: this might show me how much force had caused her death. There was no bruising.

I had to move the artery aside a little (more spiderwebs broken) to fully expose the vagus nerve. Wrapped in Schwann cells, the nerve is whiter than the carotid artery, which, when you compare the two, now looks creamy. The nerve is wire-like, at about a millimetre in diameter, slightly glistening, and it musters a certain sinuous dignity on its long journey from the base of the skull, famously, to the heart. But it does not stop there: it continues into the abdomen, finishing at the colon. The vagus nerve looks as though it would like to travel in a straight line, but it accommodates the obstruction of other bodily systems with a deferential grace by bowing where necessary into the slightest of curves.

I closely examined the area around Clare's vagus nerve for deep bruising: once again, I was searching for signs of force. Once again, I found none. The nerve looked harmless enough. But I believed it was probably responsible for the death of this child.

The vagus nerve is part of the body's autonomic system.

That means it doesn't consult us, it simply controls things we never think about, like our heartbeat. When Clare was strangled, the vagus nerve carried the message to her heart that it should slow down. Why did it give this false instruction? For the same reason that banging the funny bone in your elbow causes tingling in your little finger. When pressure was put on the vagus nerve by the ligature, the nerve became stimulated. Unlike the ulnar nerve in the elbow, the vagus nerve, when stimulated, has a fatal reflex. It slows the heart. In Clare's case, it slowed the heart so much that it stopped beating and she died.

As martial arts experts well know, a single blow to the vagus nerve can result in almost instant death, but the exact mechanism which causes this is subject to some dispute. Few American pathologists would agree with the widely held British theory of strangulation. They might argue that in fact Clare died because the ligature stimulated the sensors not around the vagus nerve but around her carotid artery. These warn the brain that blood pressure is too high, prompting the heart to slow down. Others argue that death is caused by a combination of carotid artery and vagus nerve misinformation, and a few would say that compression of the jugular vein also plays its part. Some are sure they understand why pressure on a certain place in the neck can kill within ten seconds, but all we can be certain of is that it happens. And it happened to Clare Romeril.

That she had died of compression of the neck caused by ligature strangulation was obvious. What the police were still waiting for me to tell them was: had she accidentally caught her necklace on a branch as she crawled beneath it, making her the unhappy victim of the mysterious vagal reflex which then stopped her heart? Or had someone strangled her?

There were no signs of violence or struggle. I had found no further evidence of bruising on the muscles of the neck. There were no abrasions or defence injuries to indicate the involvement of a third party. I had to leave the police's questions unanswered and the inspector gave me a look of extreme frustration as we left the post-mortem room.

Behind us, there was the usual rustle of mortuary assistants preparing to work on the body. They would now use their great talents to return Clare to the state those who loved her had known and could grieve over. The post-mortem, by definition, is an invasive procedure. It is carried out in the interests of the deceased and those left behind and, where foul play is discovered, of wider society. All post-mortems are performed with very great respect. And they are sometimes carried out more than once.

'I should probably come back in a few days,' I said. 'There's a chance that bruises are under the skin somewhere and just haven't come out yet.'

'She's dead,' the inspector said mournfully. 'The bruises aren't going to come out now.'

'I assure you,' I said, 'that they are.'

Once again, he looked sceptical. I could have argued, but I had other places to go.

4

It was morning now. There was busy traffic outside the mortuary. The police officers were all going home, but I was still wide awake and decided to take this opportunity to visit the place where Clare's body had been found.

The inspector approved of this. He said: 'My boss is there, I'll tell her you're coming.'

I drove to the park, much of which had been closed off. Blue-and-white POLICE – DO NOT CROSS tape was strung from tree to tree. In fact, although it was winter, this was a very pleasant place. Once, it had been the extensive grounds of a big country house. The house had been demolished, but its world of rolling lawns and large, shrubby borders lived on.

A detective sergeant took me through the tape.

'Find anything useful at the post-mortem?' he asked.

'Clare was strangled,' I told him.

He gave me a sidelong glance.

'We already guessed that, Doc. We all saw her neck.'

'I can't tell you much more, at this stage,' I said. He looked away. I recognized that disappointment the police always feel but don't express when the pathologist can't solve their crime for them.

He introduced me to the superintendent. She looked like a woman who'd had a good night's sleep.

'Just came on duty to this one,' she said cheerfully. 'I love my job. You never know what's going to happen when you get to work in the morning.'

'Can you give me any background on Clare Romeril?' I asked. The officers who had attended the post-mortem had supplied some of this, but I guessed that by now there would be more information and that the super would have been fully briefed before her arrival.

She told me that Clare's biological father had divorced her mother some time ago and the police had already interviewed him. He had been at a local football game the afternoon of her disappearance and then went out with other fans in the evening, so there were plenty of people to confirm that he was with them at the time of Clare's death. The investigating officers had also learned that in recent weeks there had been anger and arguments in Clare's house and that her stepfather, George Romeril, had actually left home. The evening of Clare's death, he had been at the same football game as her father and had even more friends to confirm it.

Mrs Romeril was, of course, very upset. Yes, Clare had been particularly difficult the day of her death: she'd had to reprimand her several times. Clare, evidently plotting her escape, had then announced she would like to go to bed right now. Mrs Romeril also had a younger daughter and, after putting both girls to bed in the early evening, had run a bath for herself. When she had finished her bath, she went to check on the girls. And discovered that Clare was missing.

I got out the sketch plan the dog handler had supplied.

'Shame the body was moved,' I said. 'She'd been dead for some time when she was found.'

'How long?' the super asked.

'I think she died between five and seven o'clock.'

'That early?'

'I think so. But . . .' How many times have I said this to a

68

police officer and watched their crestfallen look? '. . . time of death is very hard to estimate accurately.'

The super and I turned down a little path, ducked under more tape, and she pointed to the place Clare had been found. I turned the sketch around and around in my hand until it lined up with the scene before me.

'Are you sure it was here? Not right under the fallen tree?'

'More under the bushes, apparently.'

Those bushes showed no broken branches or any other signs of a struggle. The previous night the weather had been windy and it had rained once or twice. But there was little evidence of activity on the muddy ground where the body had lain, certainly no more foot marks than one would expect from paramedics following the path in and out.

'Aha,' I said. 'I can see where the Coke can was.'

Forensics had taken it, but its indentation on the damp earth was still clear, just as the little blue stone on Clare's necklace had left its indentation on her throat.

The weak winter sun came out. It was forensically safe for me to move around the site, and I did so now, crouching, looking at the tree and its sturdy offshoots, examining the bushes, trying to see where a low branch could have snagged that necklace. I couldn't find one.

'Seen enough?' the super asked as I returned to the path. She was trying to scrape the mud off her shoes and on to a patch of damp grass before she returned to her office. I did the same, but the mud was obstinate.

I was thinking. Something was wrong. I remembered Clare's clothes, the My Little Pony T-shirt, the skirt. The pink trainers.

I said: 'You'd hardly know Clare had been here at all.'

The super was busy with her shoes.

69

'What do you mean?'

Now I had to be careful. The police aren't always receptive to pathologists who try to tell them what to think.

'Let's suppose for a moment that Clare was killed here. How could anyone have done that without the child struggling and getting her clothes covered in mud? In particular, her shoes.'

The super looked at me closely and wrapped her coat tighter around her. The weather was dryer today, but it was just as windy.

'That's one reason we think this was an accidental death,' she pointed out. 'No struggle.'

'The necklace would have been snagged from a branch overhead. Yet, according to this sketch, she was found on her back with her hands by her sides. Not that we know that for sure, of course.'

'God, if only someone had taken a picture,' the super sighed.

'And just look at your shoes now . . .'

The super stared down again miserably. 'I've got some tissues in the car.'

'But Clare's trainers were clean,' I said.

The super looked back up at me.

'Ah, but she might have been asphyxiated as soon as she crawled in there,' she suggested. 'Then there wouldn't have been much mud on her trainers.'

'Or if she was killed somewhere else and carried here, there would have been no mud at all. Not on her trainers. Not anywhere.'

She looked thoughtful. In those days I was still of the opinion that cigarettes were an essential tool in the thinking process. So I got out a packet and offered her one. The sun appeared again and we leaned away from it to light up out of the wind and then turned back so that its warmth would touch our faces. The wind whipped away the smoke and for a moment we breathed deeply in silence. A cigarette could be relied upon to ease any sadness other people's deaths might cause. As for thinking about our own, well, smoking helped us not to do that, too. And we couldn't even see the irony.

The super began to talk about Clare's mother. Mrs Romeril was upset but perhaps not upset enough. In fact, the super had found her version of events slightly unsatisfactory. The stepfather had been out at the football match but there was a lodger in the family's flat who'd been at home with some mates the evening before, playing cards. Their statements might not stand up in court because they had been smoking a lot of marijuana and, for other reasons as well, were vulnerable at best to challenge and at worst to character assassination by a sharp defence barrister, but their stories did at least concur.

The lodger had described the fraught nature of Mrs Romeril's relationship with Clare. The child was often difficult, the mother often angry. That afternoon, both lodger and friends reported that there had been a lot of shouting and tears. When the fracas was over, Mrs Romeril had put both her daughters furiously to bed. Then she had run a bath and told the card-players that she was going to have a good soak and relax. She'd disappeared. They'd assumed she was having that bath, but when she had re-emerged, about half an hour later, all of them noticed that she had not been wearing a dressing gown or lounge clothes, as you might expect after a bath. She had fully dressed again. And she had been wearing outdoor shoes.

'Well, we've taken her shoes, so we can have them checked

for mud and pollen to see if she was in this park,' the super told me. 'There's no chance of finding a footprint worth matching here.'

Pollen doesn't just happen in the spring; it is fine as dust and present all the time. If Mrs Romeril had been in the park, then there would be mud and a pollen mix on her shoes to prove it, even in winter.

We looked at each other now. Were we saying that a mother might have killed her seven-year-old daughter? That would be so rare that it would place this case far outside the usual probabilities. Police suspicions nearly always centre on males: father or stepfather, partner, lodger or any other significant male.

'Obviously,' the super said, 'we're checking their alibis, but so far they seem pretty sound.'

But Clare's clean trainers alone, I thought, pointed to the possibility – no, the probability – of death elsewhere. And so, a homicide.

The father, the stepfather and the mother were all questioned intensively, but no arrest was made. There was simply not enough evidence.

Four days later I returned to the mortuary to examine the body a second time. This is usual in such circumstances: despite the detective's scepticism, in death, as well as in life, bruises can take some time to show. And sure enough, I found a band of discoloration across the back of Clare's neck.

The same detective was present and said: 'Yeah, I thought so. I'm sure I could see that bruise at the first post-mortem.'

I didn't dignify this with a reply. The fact was, the circle of the ligature mark was now complete: it was at the front, the side and the back of the neck. And so the case changed. It became a murder inquiry. It's one thing for a child to get a necklace caught in a bush and for it to cause so much pressure across the front of the neck that she is asphyxiated. It's another for the necklace to be wound so tightly all around the neck that the child dies. This strongly, although not conclusively, suggests human intervention.

The police had now ruled out the father, the stepfather, the lodger and the lodger's mates. But Clare's trainers had been re-examined and no mud found on them. And there were very scant traces of the pollens from the park. The soles of Mrs Romeril's shoes, however, bore dried mud and some very distinctive pollen that must indeed have come from the park because, right next to the place where Clare had been found, was a rare oak tree.

The expert from Kew was ecstatic.

'There are only a few in the whole country,' she said. 'And not another one within a hundred miles of here. Must be a remnant left by some Victorian plant-hunter who visited the big house.'

Mrs Romeril was quick to point out that, as she lived in a flat next to the park, she often went there. In fact, on the afternoon of Clare's death she had been near the rare tree with her children.

Clare's trainers did suggest that she had been killed and moved to the park, but a dead seven-year-old is quite a weight. At post-mortem she weighed 22.1 kilos and so the police began once more to consider the involvement of a man. Perhaps, when Clare had left the house with her little bag, there had been a most unfortunate encounter with a homicidal stranger.

Such an event almost always creates a press furore which terrifies every parent in the land. The chances of this happening to any child are, statistically, minimal. In the light of such wide coverage, the police were nevertheless obliged to start a manhunt, questioning all the males in the area.

'You wouldn't believe how many blokes can prove they were at that football match,' the super said wearily over the phone a few weeks later.

A second pathologist, as is usual, was called in, and by now a further bruise had appeared on Clare's body. I daresay that the know-it-all detective had noticed it at the first post-mortem, too. It was large, on the right shoulder blade, and it did seem to indicate the application of some strong pressure. Noting that the neck ligature marks extended slightly upwards behind both ears, this pathologist suggested that the ligature had been pulled from behind and forced upwards. He suggested that there had been another ligature, not necessarily the necklace. I thought it unlikely that another three-millimetre ligature had been used but agreed when he said that the assailant had been behind Clare and the child had probably been upright or semi-upright when pressure was applied.

If there had been any lingering doubt that Clare had been murdered, this discovery of further bruising eradicated it. But, despite a full investigation, the murderer remained entirely faceless. It looked as if the Clare Romeril case would remain unsolved.

Some time later, I attended the American Academy of Forensic Sciences annual conference. I cross the Atlantic for this whenever I can because it often brings me in direct contact with new ideas, new information, new ways of thinking. And old friends. We take our most interesting files and it is our pleasure to discuss them late into the night in the hotel bar. To help each other and expose our human weakness by occasionally showing off how clever we have been. On the first evening we are guarded, aware how horrifying the subject matter must be to any staff or other guests who happen to overhear it. But as the conference wears on we get more and more casual about tossing scene-of-crime pictures at each other, loudly exchanging questions, ideas, sometimes wisdom and occasionally enlightenment.

Richard Walter was a founder member of the exclusive Vidocq Society. This is a collection of distinguished detectives and forensic experts. For years they met each month to apply their considerable combined talents to cold cases presented to them by police forces who were truly stumped. Hollywood and many American newspapers have been apt to label them 'the heirs to Sherlock Holmes'.

I was sharing cases with Richard that evening and we were probably on our third glass of wine when I produced the Romeril file. I explained the circumstances and Richard looked at the file and glanced through the police reports. The bar was thick with smoke; we all smoked, and Richard perhaps more than anyone. In his hand was a menthol cigarette and a glass of white wine; he was seldom, at this stage of the evening, seen without either.

He handled the sketches and photos from the file carefully, holding them between thin, agile fingers. Richard started his career as a lab technician, then, after qualifying as a psychologist, worked in jails in Michigan, where he interviewed thousands and thousands of inmates. He has also been involved with the FBI analysis of serial murderers. He was and is one of America's foremost forensic psychologists. When he turns his gaze on me, I can find myself squirming like a lab specimen under a stark light. He has the ability, innate but honed through long experience, to read human behaviour – and not just the behaviour of offenders.

75

Now he closed the Romeril file, lit another cigarette, topped up his glass of wine.

'The police really don't know what they're looking for,' I said. 'A madman in the park or . . .'

'Or the kid's mother.'

I blinked at him in surprise. I hadn't even told him our thoughts about Mrs Romeril and how the cannabis-smoking lodgers had said they had noticed her strange choice of foot-wear immediately after her 'long soak in the bath' that night. Nor how the pollen expert had matched the mud on that footwear to a unique tree in the park.

Richard leaned towards me.

'What was in the bag?'

I paused.

'The bag?'

'The kid's bag.'

Ah, her running-away bag. I took back the file and flicked through it until I found at the back a few pages of documen-tation the police had given me. This included a list of the bag's contents, which I had never really studied before because it had seemed irrelevant.

I read out loud: 'One pair of pink socks. Two pairs of underpants, sized for age six. Green sweater. Packet of tis-sues. T-shirt, pink with glitter My Little Pony . . .'

There was a strange, deep, guttural sound. Then another. The noise was issuing from behind a large glass of white wine and it wasn't hiccoughing.

'What's so funny?' I asked. Richard was grinning broadly.

'You think a seven-year-old kid packs that stuff? She's leaving home, right? So she takes her favourite plastic horse, the one with the purple mane. And the barrette that fell out of a Christmas cracker. And the yellow cup and saucer from

Barbie's tea set. Except she can't fit the cup in so she just takes the saucer. And that little box with the shells on. And a pink glitter pen. That's how a kid packs her bag.'

I knew he was right. Once, when my daughter was small and our holiday was over, she'd announced that she was all packed and ready to go. Her suitcase turned out to be full of the beach, including seaweed, sand and a wellington boot.

I tried to imagine the small girl I had examined in the post-mortem room busily and sensibly finding clean socks and pants to put in her running-away bag. Ridiculous. Impossible.

'Whoever packed that bag for the kid killed her,' Richard said. 'In my opinion.'

He drained the wine and lit another cigarette. My round, I thought. But I did not move.

'She was probably grabbed by the necklace from behind . . .' I said slowly. It was like feeding a voracious fire. I knew he would soon burn up this piece of information.

'Okay, so the mother's getting mad at the kid and, instead of looking contrite, the kid just turns and walks away. That is so damn annoying for a parent. The mother walks after the kid and grabs at her. She gets the necklace. Maybe she means to kill her, maybe she doesn't, maybe she wants to stop her walking off and just hurt her a bit. But suddenly Mom's got a vagus reflex on her hands and a dead daughter.'

My eyes were fixed on the orange glow at the end of his cigarette. I couldn't possibly address this without lighting one myself.

'You don't think it was deliberate?'

'It might have been.'

'But if it wasn't, and she suddenly realized Clare was dead, the mother must have . . . ?' I was still way behind him.

'Does she try to resuscitate her?' His face stretched into

an eerie, yellow-toothed smile. 'No. She thinks fast. Quick decision, she goes for a cover-up.'

'You mean . . . her daughter's dead at her feet and she decides to make it look as if she's run away? And immediately packs that bag? And tells the lodger she's having a bath? And turns on the taps . . . ?'

'And then carries the girl and the bag not very far at all, because the kid's a deadweight, remember . . .'

'Hoping no one sees her?'

'It's winter, it's dark, and didn't you say everyone's at a ball game?'

Yes. The super had said it seemed that the whole housing estate was there.

'She shoves her under a bush in the park and, if her DNA's all over the kid, well, it would be, she's Mom.'

'That shows . . . a certain presence of mind,' I said. 'If she really didn't plan to kill Clare.'

'Yup. This woman has the intelligence and quick thinking of a master criminal or a captain of industry.'

I thought of the Romerils' ugly seventies flat, which the super had shown me from the outside. It had shouted hopelessness and deprivation. Who would have thought the place could house such a mighty brain?

Now Richard reached for a file of his own.

'Okay,' he said, 'your turn. Small island, scattered farming community. Fourteen-year-old girl walking home from a church meet-up. Local guy finds bloodstains on the road the next morning, but no body. Police search eventually discovers the body of a young girl, a hundred yards away, up a hillside. Raped. Bloodstained rock beside her head. But no blood spatter on the ground.' He threw me a set of photos. 'Work this one out, Dick.'

78

When I got back to the UK, I phoned the super.

'Clare Romeril, yeah,' she said wearily. Clare was many cases ago now and the super had reached that stage where she just wanted the file off her desk.

I told her what Richard Walter had suggested.

'God!' There was a long pause. 'Well. You say this Richard's an eminent psychologist and it . . . it really sounds as though he's right. About the bag. About all of it. We've interviewed the mother and interviewed her again, but let's get her in once more. The trouble is, we can't prove any of it unless she cracks. And your friend's correct: she's a smart cookie. There's never enough evidence on this one for the Crown Prosecution Service.'

And there never was enough evidence. To this day, no one has been arrested for Clare's murder. At the inquest, the coroner returned a verdict of unlawful killing. Aware of newspaper reports that the mother had been interviewed many times, he told the court that he could not entertain the possibility that she had killed her seven-year-old daughter in cold blood. Mrs Romeril was exonerated.

However, it was not long before I heard from the local authority. They wanted to remove Clare's younger sister from Mrs Romeril's care and were asking me to give evidence to the family court. Their case was successful. Although there was never enough evidence to convict her of homicide beyond reasonable doubt, the family court uses a lower level of proof and so took the view that, on the balance of probabilities, she had been involved in Clare's death – or anyway had been implicated in her death. Her surviving daughter was removed to be kept safe from her.

This case tells us so much about unnatural death in childhood. Behind it, as so often, there is a deprived and troubled family history and the victim is a child whose welfare depends on a parent who is lacking the resources or skills – although, in this case, certainly not the intelligence – to cope. And Clare's case teaches us something of our own attitude to childhood and parenting. We expect children to start encountering the world by the time they are seven. Despite our best endeavours, we know that occasionally the consequences of this exploration can be tragic.

Statistically, homicide does not even appear among the major causes of death for girls of this age (boys are a different matter), but accidents are relatively common. And how willing we were at first to call Clare's death an accident. After that, how ready the newspapers were to believe that she had run out of her home alone and been abducted by a stranger. In 2007, three-year-old Madeleine McCann was snatched by a stranger from a holiday resort in Portugal and, at the time of writing, German police have identified a paedophile as the very likely suspect. A few years earlier, eight-year-old Sarah Payne was grabbed by a convicted sex offender when she was playing outside her grandparents' house in rural Sussex: her body was found weeks later in a shallow grave.

Abductions by complete strangers, as in Sarah Payne's case and perhaps Madeleine McCann's, almost always involve sexual motivation. However, Clare had not been sexually assaulted or raped. We know abuse, sexual or otherwise, to be statistically much more likely to come from inside the family than outside. We perceive the threat, but we perceive it as male. Indeed, the statistical likelihood of a mother killing her child (although mothers are recognized as killers of babies) is minuscule. And it is almost impossible for us to see mothers as child-killers. I believe this, plus her strong sense of self-preservation and sharp wits, ensured that Mrs Romeril did not face trial for Clare's death.

The fates of Clare Romeril, Sarah Payne and perhaps Madeleine McCann are shocking but should not greatly overshadow other childhoods. I re-emphasize their rarity. After that dangerous first year of life, the chances of dying in childhood plummet by more than 95 per cent. By the time the child is around the age of four, congenital abnormalities have probably already shown themselves and there is less susceptibility to infectious disease. Result: the ages between five and nine are the safest across an entire lifetime, with ages between ten and fourteen not far behind.

How, then, do children die? Well, there is of course the risk of infection: meningitis, sepsis and, increasingly, measles, can still be deadly. Infectious diseases accounted in 2018 for about 6 per cent of child deaths. Accidents and the untoward accounted for about 15 per cent, perhaps because curiosity, as the child grows, may exceed an understanding of risk, but more often because children are vulnerable pedestrians and cyclists. Cars, however, are not the greatest child-killer. Cancer is, by far. Childhood cancer has been steadily increasing, worldwide, since the 1960s, rising by about 11 per cent between 2000 and 2017.

Reporting and diagnosis has certainly improved since the 1960s, but that cannot really explain such dramatic figures. There is broad agreement on only one thing: the cause may well be at least partly environmental, reflecting some aspect of our modern lives, perhaps chemicals or technology, which we wrongly regard as harmless.

The commonest childhood cancer is acute lymphoblastic leukaemia. This is the over-production of white blood cells in the bone marrow, a sorcerer's apprentice of a process by which uselessly immature white cells are produced uncontrollably. They crowd out the normal red and white blood cells as well as the little cells that help clotting – platelets – thus causing the first and most obvious symptoms, bruising and anaemia.

Leukaemia is not regarded as hereditary, although there may sometimes be hereditary factors. We simply don't know what causes most cases. Researchers have made the interesting observation that children who were in day care during their first year are less likely to develop leukaemia: they have been exposed to the coughs, colds, viruses and bacteria of a communal environment. While sufferers, as babies, were probably largely isolated from infection.

A detailed study now proposes that exposure to infection early in life may be protective. Our immune systems need 'priming', a way of learning what is out there, so that, when the same infections are encountered a little later, they are dealt with much more swiftly. This, of course, is the main principle behind vaccination, and there is now some evidence that the routine early childhood vaccinations may also offer some protection against leukaemia. This cancer may result from a combination of factors – genes, diet, luck, or some other variable we don't know about. But if Western society's pristine, modern houses represent a behavioural change, then perhaps our immune systems are missing the peck of dirt of yesteryear.

The same theory is currently applied by some doctors to our soaring rates of asthma. This is a disease that is caused by an incorrectly functioning immune system and one for which over a million children in the UK are receiving treatment (about one in eleven, according to Asthma UK). Data is variable but we know, even if the incidence is levelling out, that taking increased population size into account, at least three times as many children now have asthma diagnosed as in the 1960s. The hygiene theory brings hope to asthmatic children and their parents (as well as to anyone who hates housework), but it is particularly encouraging to those suffering from leukaemia. It suggests that changes in our approach to immunity may mean childhood's biggest monster can be slain.

And then the lover;
Sighing like furnace, with a woeful ballad
Made to his mistress' eyebrow:

5

It was summer, but my holidays were over and it was back to the dark world of sudden and unnatural deaths. I had been planning to ease myself in gently with a morning's flying. This is my own private escape. I have always been in love with the idea of cutting free from gravity and the ties of earthly existence, of slicing through thin air high above the world. But it never seemed possible that I would actually fly an aircraft myself. Then, one day, thanks to the Metropolitan Police flying club, to my own amazement I was able to do just that.

While other people, when there is a clear blue sky and a light breeze, might think of beaches or moors or hills, I had been dreaming of only one thing that Sunday – flying through the blueness behind the controls of a small aircraft. But the day had dawned grey, the weather was foul and the flight I had been longing for was off. So, when the police contacted me to go to a camping site near a distant beauty spot, I seized the chance of a little solitude on the journey and set off at once.

It was August, but the weather had been sent by winter and, as the unseasonal storm raged in from the Atlantic, I reminded myself of that old aviation saying: it is much better to be looking up at the sky wishing you were there than down on the ground wishing the same. Rain and wind buffeted the car on the main roads as I headed towards the countryside and, later, on the back lanes, I twice got out to move aside fallen branches, heavy with wet summer leaves.

The campsite was little more than a sheltered field on a farm and it had almost no facilities. Evidently, entry was restricted to just a few tents, as only a couple of these were pitched. They were far apart, at the very corners of the field. On the other hand, there might have been more campers before the arrival of bad weather, police cars, tracker dogs, forensic teams, journalists and, now, a pathologist, none of these being conducive to a happy holiday.

Attention was focused on a small, blue tent in the far corner, which had tape all around it, curving and flapping in the gale. The police had made a narrow entry-and-exit path to the tent to keep footfall around it as contained as possible.

An officer was trying to drive her police car out through the gate, but by now the field was poached by the traffic and a couple more officers had to push her. The car roared as its wheels fought with the mud. Everyone looked cold and wet. I parked my car at a distance, where the ground seemed firm.

I know that driving an elderly Volvo Estate means I could be mistaken for an antiques dealer, and a shady one at that, but how many cars can you open up at the back and sit in to pull on a Tyvek suit? A detective inspector arrived and introduced himself while I did this. He was already covered from the head down in white. And he wore the special bootees the police are also supplied with.

'It's wellingtons for me,' I told him, reaching for mine. He looked envious.

I realize I may have given the impression that homicide scenes are always seas of mud because the cases I have chosen for this book may be misleading in that respect. Most crime scenes are in built-up areas and the white bootees with POLICE stamped on the sole are usually adequate. Not today, though. The DI's bootees were not bearing up well to the rigours of the camping field.

'Girl's dead inside. We're looking for the boyfriend,' he said, as we headed off for the tent. He paused while a deafening police helicopter swung low overhead, skittering around just below the clouds. I was jealous of the pilot for flying today, although I knew this must be a bouncy ride. The photographer taking the overviews wouldn't be enjoying it at all.

The detective eventually shouted over the noise: 'They were last seen outside the tent on Friday evening, so he could have got a long way.'

'When was she found?' I asked.

'This afternoon. The weather was dry on Friday night; people saw them sitting outside, talking and eating. Then, on Saturday, there's nothing happening but no one's watching, no one cares. Today someone thought it was a bit odd that their tent was still shut up and their bikes were still chained to the gate over there . . .'

'They came here by bike?' I asked, surprised. A cycling and camping holiday was the sort of budget vacation my parents took when they were young. In the late 1930s, they had cycled all around northern France on a tandem, so much in love that they had noticed little but each other: the journal they kept fails to note the imminent outbreak of war.

'Well, these two don't live far away,' the detective said. 'They go to a local school.'

'You've got their names?'

'Yep, got their phones. She's sixteen, he's seventeen, and we think he killed her.'

Teenage boy kills teenage girl is rare enough. And as I crossed the field in my wellies, watching the DI's shoes emerge through the useless white bootees and his trousers getting wetter and wetter at the ankle, I thought how murder and camping holidays were an incongruous combination. However, the detective seemed confident and my job has taught me that homicide, although sometimes drearily predictable, is also likely to be full of surprises.

As we reached the tent, I put on my mask and gloves. One tent flap had been secured open but, despite this fresh air, I noticed as I crawled into the space beside the body that the atmosphere in here was tired and stale. The air had an acidic edge.

The dead girl's face was pink, her skin unlined, her cheeks childishly rounded. Dark hair tumbled to the ground. How often had I looked down at my own daughter, asleep and safe at home? But this girl was not asleep.

The sleeping bag had been cut back from her body by the paramedics and their detritus now littered the ground. I examined her carefully. If this couple had come here with sexual intentions, the cold seemed to have intercepted them. She was wearing a thick pair of pyjamas, socks and a sweater. I looked for any wounds which had penetrated her clothing. There were none. And I found no bloodstains. The lower half of her body was well covered, the pyjamas tucked in beneath the upper band of a pair of underpants, so there was no indicator yet of violent or unwelcome sexual activity.

It was impossible for me to stand up in the tent. I continued to kneel by the girl's side as I looked around. A few feet away was a second sleeping bag. You could easily see where someone had climbed out of it, leaving it ball-shaped. A backpack. A few clothes and a jumble of trainers. They had not been worn since the weather had deteriorated; the absence of mud told me that. And, in the corner, a silver tray

filled with dark ash: the remains of a cheap, disposable barbecue. I shuffled backwards out of the tent.

The detective inspector and his colleagues were waiting
for me at a distance, nearer the field entrance, in the lee of a
CSI van.

I took off my gloves and mask.

'It was fine on Friday night, but I think it was quite cold?'
I asked. We had arrived home that evening from our sunny
holiday and it had seemed arctic to us when we landed. All
the detectives nodded.

'I took my kids swimming at the outdoor pool, but they
wouldn't go in,' one said.

'Got any idea how he did it?' the DI asked me.

I opened my mouth to speak but saw that a junior officer
was trying to catch my eye. It was obvious she was bursting
to say something.

'Doc . . . is it anything to do with the barbecue?'

I nodded.

The junior detective looked around at her colleagues. She
did not actually say the words 'I told you so!' but her face
spoke for her.

'I think you're probably right,' I said. God knows how the
couple had carried that tray of charcoal here on their bikes.
Maybe the farmer had sold it to them, or they had picked it
up at the village shop I had passed a mile or so back. 'Obviously, I'll need to have a close look at post-mortem, but at
this point I'd say they may have taken the barbecue into the
tent to help them keep warm and –'

'Carbon monoxide poisoning!' The young detective simply
could not contain herself. I nodded.

There are some bosses who are delighted when juniors do

something clever and there are some who simply resent it, and this woman's boss fell into the latter category.

'Then how do you explain the fact,' he said, icily, looking only at me, 'that she died and he didn't?'

Carbon monoxide is a strange gas, and it is deadly. In fact, it is odourless, so some years ago suppliers used to add a nasty onion odour to the coal gas then used for domestic supply, so that it was easy to smell leaks (and the same is true of modern natural gas, even though there is no carbon monoxide in it). What makes CO poisonous is its love of haemoglobin. It clings to this critical chemical in our red blood cells at least 250 times more strongly than the oxygen the cells should be transporting. So any carbon monoxide in the atmosphere displaces oxygen in the blood, potentially accumulating until the blood is carrying mainly CO. The body's tissues then become starved of oxygen. Even tiny amounts of CO in the atmosphere – as low as 0.1 per cent – can mean that the level in the blood reaches a fatal point within a couple of hours. And higher concentrations – for instance, from the exhaust of a car engine left running in a small garage with the doors closed – can kill in less than ten minutes.

Personal sensitivity to the saturation of carbon monoxide in the blood varies greatly. A concentration of 50 per cent in the blood will be fatal for most healthy adults – but not all. And older people or those with arterial or respiratory diseases will certainly succumb earlier than the young and fit. In the days when coal gas appliances were poorly regulated (and, unfortunately, this is still the case in holiday villas in some countries), whole rooms of people were occasionally found dead from CO poisoning. Often, they showed wildly differing saturation levels.

The symptoms are stealthy. Some victims may experience nothing stronger than a headache and slight nausea before lapsing into a coma and dying. At about 40 per cent saturation, they may be very nauseous, probably vomiting, feeling weak and sinking towards a coma, while at 30 per cent saturation, they may just appear drunk.

I explained this to the police officers, and one soon had his notebook open.

'A couple walked right past these two on the way back from the caves, just when it was getting dark. And one of them said . . .' Flick, flick. The policeman read the walker's words flatly: '"I thought they were daft for letting their fire go out, they both looked so chilly. But they were having a bit of a row and didn't seem to notice."'

'Why did they bring it in, then? If it was out and wasn't going to keep them warm?' someone asked.

'In case it got wet?' the eager junior suggested. 'They might have wanted to use it again.'

'But surely if the fire was out, it couldn't have killed them,' another officer said.

'A charcoal fire can look as if it's finished but still be burning slowly and producing carbon monoxide,' I said.

The junior was bursting to speak again.

'The boy must have known that!' She turned to one of her colleagues. 'Didn't you say he was doing science A-levels? He might have known how dangerous it was and that the fumes would kill her. Bet he waited for her to fall asleep and then got himself out quickly.'

Her boss did not look at her. He just rolled his eyes.

I said: 'Alternatively, there's a chance he woke up very befuddled by fumes, couldn't wake her and stumbled off into the night to get help. Carbon monoxide poisoning makes people feel very ill and it also makes them behave in strange ways.'

The DI shook his head. 'His head would have cleared once he was outside, though. Right, Doc?'

It was possible that, if the boy had only a headache and felt sick and confused, his symptoms would have gradually eased when he was away from the fumes in the cool night air. But that would take a while. On the other hand, his brain could have been so deprived of oxygen that it would never recover from the damage.

'If he was well enough to walk away, he was well enough to phone the police!' the DI insisted. 'Instead of which, he's gone off, God knows where, left his bike, left his clothes. Left her.'

There was no point arguing. It was essential to find the boy, and the officer obviously had no intention of halting either manhunt or murder inquiry.

The forensic team had completed their work and I watched as they put the girl, still snug in her floral sleeping bag, into another bag: a harsh white body bag. He zipped it up. A CSI wrote 'Unknown Female – Frenchay Farm' in felt pen on the outside. I asked the coroner's officer to transfer the girl's body to the local mortuary for post-mortem as soon as possible. And a short time later the DI stood next to me in his wet feet and wet trousers and we watched the body bag being slid into the hearse. I felt sure he was hoping that when we saw the body in the mortuary there would be signs of strangulation or something similar to confirm his theory. And I was pretty certain that I would find none.

I was soon to hear from him again. I had just changed into my scrubs in the mortuary and was wondering where he'd got to when my phone rang.

He did not greet me.

'Okay, Doc, we've found the boy!'

'Great, where is he?'

'At the quarry. It's just nearby.'

'What's he saying?'

There was a pause.

'He's dead.'

I wished I hadn't already changed into my scrubs.

'You haven't started on the girl yet, have you?' he asked.

'No, I was waiting for you.'

'Can you come and take a look at him right now?'

'How far away is the quarry?'

'It's in the woods right behind the campsite. Looks as though he killed her then topped himself.'

Of course, once I had changed back into my clothes, I had to explain the delay to the waiting mortuary assistants. They were on overtime and so were delighted to retreat for tea, chocolate biscuits and an afternoon romcom on the TV while I went back to the campsite.

I did so with a slight sense of disquiet. The police were very keen to turn what seemed like a tragic accident into foul play.

By now the track was a mud bath. I drove as slowly as I could as far as I could and then slid gracefully to a halt. Wellies back on, I squelched to the CSI van.

The DI was waiting for me once again. He led me up the field, past the tent where the girl's body had lain, through a small gate. There was a narrow track here and the woods were thick and quite dark. He was wearing a new pair of white bootees over his shoes, which I could see were unlikely to last much longer.

After about 300 metres, we stopped. He pointed to his right, down a barely trodden path with police markers on either side.

'We think he went down that track, so we'll have to go straight on.'

We continued, brushing against foliage, to the edge of a sandstone cliff. On the left, the track turned and descended. On the right was a small picnic area, its boundaries defined by a line of blue tape, whipping in the wind that roared up the cliff face.

The woods here were a local attraction because they were full of such cliffs and some had caves which, right up to the beginning of the twentieth century, had still been lived in. Now the only inhabitants were the forensic team, who were on their hands and knees, searching. Their faces, as they gestured us through, spoke volumes, and those volumes did not include the word 'happy'.

This area had been created as a viewing site. The grass had been cut recently and was short and spiky. There was a picnic table with fixed benches and, between any picnickers and the cliff edge, was only one large log. Above, trees now sheltering us from the rain would have provided some shade on most August days and, if you looked straight ahead, you should have been able to see for miles across the countryside. Except today, low grey clouds were hurling themselves towards us. Trees, growing from below, swayed at eye level, birds huddling in their branches. Definitely not a day to go flying. And not a day to stand on a cliff, either.

'CSI tell me that he hung about and smoked a few cigarettes,' the officer said.

Even now a photographer was taking pictures of bruised grass and a small pile of cigarette butts.

'Then I think he jumped. You can see where he went over the edge, here . . .'

Yes, I could see that the cliff edge had been disturbed and

that, on its very lip, sandstone was visible which had recently been exposed.

'You'd better take a look down if you're okay with heights.'

I was so okay with heights that I had hoped to be looking down from 3,000 feet today. I stepped forward. The cliff felt solid: it must be strong, or there would surely have been more than a log to keep people back.

Not so far beneath us – I was perhaps fifty feet up – was some scrub and, beneath the bushes, white ghosts moved. Another forensic team at work.

At the centre of their activity, half obscured by foliage, face down, was a spread-eagled body. Obviously, it was a young man. He lay quite close to the cliff. His arms were twisted and his legs were splayed unevenly. A black ponytail flew out to one side of his head, as if he were still falling through the air.

We made our way between trees back to the main track and followed it down. Its serpiginous route had been designed for buggies or wheelchairs, but eventually it took us to the right level, where some blue tape marked the approved route through the undergrowth. We were now at the base of the cliff. To one side, about halfway up its sheer face, was a hollowed area that could have been a cave.

I looked from the boy's body to the cave. Was it possible that the lad had decided to scramble down the cliff face to reach it?

Again, on with gloves and mask. Again, the approach to the body. But this time the deceased looked less peaceful: he was twisted and distorted and there was heavy bloodstaining around him. I checked his fingernails. They weren't broken and there was no sandstone grime beneath them which might have indicated either that he had tried to scale the rock face or that he had made a desperate attempt to break his descent.

'He jumped, didn't he? No chance he fell?' asked the officer, watching me.

I winced and said nothing because that is one mystery medicine can seldom solve with certainty. And in the absence of an answer from me, the detective supplied his own.

'If he stopped to have a smoke first, then I think we can assume he jumped.'

He was probably right. It would be unusual to smoke at a cliff edge and then fall off it afterwards. But not impossible, especially with a head full of carbon monoxide in the dark.

'Here's the scenario as I see it,' the detective said. 'Lad gets in the tent with the girl and the cold barbecue. Says he has to bring it in because rain's forecast. Once she's asleep, he gets out fast because he knows what's going to happen. He comes into the woods to sit and think and have a cigarette. Then he jumps.'

'You really think it's a murder-suicide.'

'Yup.'

'That's one possibility,' I admitted. 'Here's another. He and the girl go into the tent and they're very cold so they bring the barbecue in as it has a bit of heat left in it. He wakes in the night, but he can't wake the girl. He's also got bad carbon monoxide poisoning and he's seriously befuddled. Maybe they had a bit of a fight and now he thinks he might have killed her because he's confused and he can't remember anything. He stumbles off into the woods . . . and falls down the cliff.'

The officer looked beady.

'Then why did he sit here smoking?'

'Do we know for sure those cigarette butts are his?'

'Forensics will prove it, but we've found a ciggy packet in his pocket, Doc.'

There was nothing for it but to get the boy in for post-mortem – although I had a feeling the two young bodies would be keeping some of their secrets hidden today.

We reconvened at the mortuary for an update, police officers filling the small meeting room, the table littered with mugs of tea, the DI uncomfortable in wet shoes.

'Okay,' said one officer who had just arrived. 'Had some interesting interviews about this pair. Let's start with Jay. His parents are definitely well off, the dad's very high up in a pharmaceutical company, his mum's a pharmacist. He's an only child and does well at school. The girl, Amelia, comes from a big family and both her parents are teachers; her dad's a deputy head. By all accounts, the boy was crazy about her. The word "obsessed" came up more than once. For instance, he had a picture of her and printed copies until he could fill one whole bedroom wall with them. And on Facebook . . .'

'Oh, no, we don't want to hear about the Devil's Window,' the DI said. 'What did she tell her mates about him?'

'Bright kid, apparently. She fell for him big time back in September, but her best friend says Amelia was finding the relationship a bit claustrophobic now. Suggestion that she thought she was pregnant – you'll be able to tell us about that, Doc.'

Not necessarily. Not if conception had occurred very recently. But the officer did not pause and I was pleased to remain silent. This team was, I feared, about to discover quite enough about the limits of forensic medicine.

'Anyway, her mates say she wanted out of the relationship; he was getting scary and possessive and she liked another kid in her class. They arranged this camping trip weeks ago because their parents were both away. She thought she couldn't really cancel so planned to use it to start breaking the news gently.' He looked up and said to no one in particular: 'Not sure that worked, really.'

The boss was nodding. It was all supporting his theory.

I looked around at their empty mugs and realized someone was missing.

'Where's that bright DC of yours?' I asked the boss.

There was a brief pause. 'She's been put on another case.'

I made no comment but stood up.

'Let's do it then,' I said. 'I gather Mum and Dad are coming to formally ID Amelia soon, so we'll start with the lad.'

They nodded and we trooped off to change.

6

Jay was ready for us in the post-mortem room and I examined his body carefully for external injuries and, of course, signs of carbon monoxide poisoning. The commonest indication among Caucasians is one which can easily be mistaken for good health: pink skin. In fact, I'd just had a holiday in the sun and I fear that for the first couple of days my own face was not dissimilar to the cherry pink which severe CO poisoning can cause.

Jay was not cherry pink; in fact, he was not pink at all. Of course, I took blood samples to establish the concentration of the gas in his blood but, from looking at him, I could not guess at the result. He had been lying on his front and so, at death, the red blood cells had drifted that way, causing the normal skin discoloration we call hypostasis. It seemed to me that this discoloured skin looked a bit brighter and pinker than one might expect. But we would have to wait for the blood analysis to be sure.

Much more obvious were the two areas of injury. They showed me that he had bounced off the cliff face on his front and left side during his descent, before the final face-down impact. I also found fractures in his left arm and both legs.

Before I opened his body to see how many organs had been ruptured, the photographer took photos of his scratched, bruised young face.

I looked at him with great compassion. Seventeen is a gawky age. Jay was tall and very skinny and his facial features were as yet rather unformed. I thought that if he had lived a few more years he would probably have grown into a handsome man. He had been deeply in love, the sort of love which marks the move from childhood to adulthood. How overpowering that first experience can be, and how ill equipped are some people, still more child than adult, to manage its excesses. Of course, no pathologist has ever succeeded in finding evidence of love in the human heart. For a physiological explanation, we must look south, towards the abdomen, to love's insistent twin: sex.

After establishing that Jay's liver and heart had been fatally ruptured by his fall, I proceeded to his male generative organs. This is a routine examination which we always carry out. Since the inside of the body is far too hot for male sexual organs, the testes descend to the scrotum around the eighth month in the womb – or, if not, then usually soon after birth. Sexual development has been measured since the 1960s on the Tanner Scale, which defines external primary and secondary characteristics. Specifically, breast size, testicular volume and pubic hair. This is a very broad guide, since everyone develops at slightly differing rates, usually but certainly not always maturing between the ages of eleven and seventeen. My own eyes, as well as the Tanner scale, told me that Jay had reached sexual maturity.

There was a deep laceration on the left side of his lower abdomen. It exposed a small section of the body's glittering, translucent packaging. I opened the tube of white, folded tissues. Inside, I uncovered, as so often in the body's packages, a bundle of vessels. Nestling together was not just the usual grouping, which consists of two vessels and a nerve. Here there was a vein, an artery and a nerve, yes . . . but also the thin rope that is the vas deferens.

Sperm are made and stored in the testes, and they are always at the ready. When orgasm is imminent, muscle contractions push them up to the prostate via the vas deferens. This is a substantial tube, about 1.5 mm in diameter, and it reminds me of a pipe-cleaner, the sort my father used to give me when I was a child to bend into animal shapes. Those pipe-cleaners had soft, fuzzy exteriors, and the vas deferens most definitely does not: it is smooth and white. But it does have a unique, tactile mixture of firmness and flexibility. Even with my eyes shut, I'd be able to identify it.

Each testis has its own vas deferens and these curve in front of the pelvic bone and pass through the folds of the peritoneum, which lines the abdominal cavity. It was here, in the inguinal space, that Jay's laceration had exposed it, sweeping up to the prostate gland. Ah, the prostate. A young man this age hardly knows or cares about his prostate. If he lives for another forty years or so, he probably becomes all too aware of it; most of us do.

The prostate sits under the bladder and produces seminal fluid. Semen is slightly anti-microbial to protect the sperm and it contains some salts and sugars to sustain them for their onward journey. That journey has already been impressively uphill through the vas deferens; now the sperm have to work even harder as the orgasmic tsunami of the seminal fluid takes them down the urethra, through the penis and into the vagina. Once there, they have to find the cervix to get to the uterus and, finally, the Fallopian tube as they strive towards their ultimate target: the egg. Think of salmon leaping upriver.

Driven ever onwards, sperm are little DNA torpedoes, well designed to swim against the female mucus flow in the race to get to the egg first. There is no second place in this sport. There are often about 200 million sperm in each milli-litre of an ejaculation, and each ejaculation is between 2 ml and 8 ml. So that's about 1,000 million sperm ready to go. But very few indeed, perhaps as few as half a dozen, actually get as far as the correct Fallopian tube.

I see fertilization as a bare-knuckle contest, a race for the egg in which there are no rules, just pure power and speed. But with a little chance along the way. Here is Dar-winian theory at its most basic – and the strongest, fittest and fastest sperm win. Small sperm, slow sperm, sperm with no tails, sperm which get lost somewhere in the cer-vical mucous, sperm which swim the wrong way or into the wrong Fallopian tube . . . all losers. Not a hope in hell of crossing the winning line first. There are very few left at the front of the race when, at last, one fuses with the egg. Immediately, changes in the egg's membrane prevent pene-tration by any further sperm and the intense competition is over.

A woman may be born with all her eggs ready for the pro-cess of monthly release, but a man makes sperm continually from puberty to death. That crucial evolutionary happening, meiosis, which happens for women in Grandma's womb, is the process which halves DNA and slightly scrambles it in preparation for a unique new person. In men, meiosis ensures that 1,000 million sperm are not just ready and (usually) able but that, incredibly, each one is genetically slightly different.

Sperm manufacture takes about three months and depends on the presence of adequate male hormones. At any one time there are billions, even zillions, at various stages of development. The production line may be buzzing in some-one of Jay's age but, once set to go, sperm have a limited shelf life. They wait in the testes for the call and, if sexual inactivity means the call has not come within a couple of weeks, they start to degrade. What to do with this potential oversupply? The thrifty body recycles them. They are broken down into their chemical components and re-used. Possibly to make new sperm. Or perhaps skin. Or maybe fingernails.

Jay's prostate was enviably compact; the size of a golf ball, as it should be. It looked strong and healthy, with none of the lumpiness which can develop as a man ages in irregular stages (ageing is certainly not a smooth process).

The prostate is directly below the bladder, which I now opened to check for any irregularities. It is a pale pink balloon, composed of interweaving bands of strong muscle, the fibres criss-crossed. The bladder feels solid and, although it can be cut with scissors, a jab with the forceps will not penetrate its thick wall. This firmness makes handling it unlike handling that other busy, muscular organ, the heart. The heart has a soft right side and a slightly firmer left side, but the bladder feels readier for mean streets than does any part of the gentle heart.

The exit route for urine from the body is the same as the exit route for sperm: the urethra. This thin pipe runs down from the bladder, right through the middle of the prostate and then onwards to the penis. It's easy to see why any trouble in the prostate means the first casualty is the bladder. If there is an obstruction, then the bladder has to work harder to expel urine and, inevitably, with such extra effort, it becomes distended.

What obstruction could there be in the prostate? About one in three men will eventually experience some enlargement of this gland, an enlargement great enough to compress the urethra running through it and block the exit of urine. This is bad plumbing design. One in eight men, and I am one of those, is diagnosed with a less benign enlargement: prostate cancer.

The young man before me now had not lived long enough to face such problems. In fact, even in death, even so badly broken, Jay's entire body rejoiced in its youth and hinted at the life which should have followed. Was his death a terrible accident or was there something more sinister, as the police believed? When such sudden, dramatic deaths occur in the young, it is hard to escape the conclusion that this was the end point of an intense personal crisis.

How lucky I was, as a teenager, to have happened across a book on forensic pathology which showed me my way in life. I knew I must do well at school to reach even the first milestone in this career: entry to medical school. I did not want to be deflected from my purpose and tried as hard as I could to steer my boat close to shore. Was it my mother's death that made me cautious? Luck? Ambition? Had something of my father's belief in the importance of education rubbed off on me? (He was immensely proud to be the first from a large and working-class family to study for a degree.) Or perhaps it was my great love, or even my great fear, of this man, who had brought me up almost alone – love and fear can coexist – which made me want to behave well and please him as much as I could.

I looked at Jay again and a certain voltage ran through me, the low but persistent voltage of old pain remembered. That sense of crisis. His sharp, young face. He reminded me not of myself as a young man but of someone else. Simon. My best friend at school.

Simon was like a colt as a teenager, all legs and arms and never quite sure what to do with them. He excelled at the exams of the day, O-levels, almost effortlessly, and then glided on towards A-levels.

His mother was a doctor and his father an engineer at a time when having two professional working parents was quite unusual. His grandmother lived with them to look after Simon and his sister. I was often at his house and loved it because it was the opposite of ours: there were shelves overflowing with books, and curiosities and family pictures were stuffed into the crevices. Nobody seemed to bother much if the place wasn't spotless. The heating was always on in winter, so there was no shivering in front of a five-bar fire. Simon was allowed to put vinyl on the hi-fi whenever he liked, and we listened as we lounged on comfortable sofas.

How sparse our house felt when I returned home from my friend's. My much older siblings had left and I was alone with my father now . . . and my stepmother. My father, in later life, confided that he still had no idea why he had married Joyce. My brother, my sister and I wondered that, too.

Before Joyce's arrival we had reached some kind of equilibrium without my mother. Initially, with my sister married and gone, it was a male sort of household with lots of spaces, the sort of spaces which women usually fill. My mother was ill throughout so much of my life that I can't pretend the house had bubbled with vibrancy and colour when she was alive – although my siblings assured me that once she had been the embodiment of vibrancy and colour. No, there was always an emptiness and, if anything filled it, then it was her illness. An illness that, unknown to me, carried a possibility. One everyone avoided talking about. That she might die.

When she did die, the spaces in the house got much bigger. My stepmother was never unpleasant or unkind, but I see now that Joyce just did not know how to be with children, particularly bereaved children, particularly boys. I think she found engaging with me so challenging that she preferred to become wallpaper. So she was there but not there. I believe I rubbed along fairly amicably with her, as though she were a live-in housekeeper. But I certainly wasn't keen to bring any friends home.

There was very often tension between Joyce and my father, which made the house's silences hum with hurt and anger. Once, when the hum became unbearable, she went home to her mother in Devon. I walked from room to room, rejoicing in the different quality of the silence. I flopped in the armchairs, picking things up and putting them down and generally reclaiming something that no one had ever taken away from me. Then, perhaps when he considered enough time had passed, my father fetched her back. I daresay he was hoping for a different outcome this time. But the cycle just began again.

Simon's house was a much nicer place to be because it was not just physically but emotionally warmer. It was full of chatter and laughter and I resolved that this was the sort of home I would strive for when I became a father. And, many years later, I did. When we had children, our house soon bore all the hallmarks of the busy middle classes of that period: daily newspapers, subscriptions to *National Geographic* and *Scientific American*, active talk at family mealtimes about politics, art and science, as well as, of course, medicine. And, as a parent, I had something else in common with Simon's parents. The importance of academic success as a route to a fulfilling career was an assumption which formed part of the architecture of our family, the way London's bus routes are built into the heart of the city.

And then the edifice fell apart for Simon. He failed his A-levels.

His parents were astonished. Shocked. No, I think they

were actually devastated. How could this have happened? He was supposed to sail through to the grades he needed to become a doctor. A place was waiting for him to study medicine at University College London.

Simon had failed so spectacularly that his parents immediately booked him into a crammer.

'What were you doing in your room every evening if not studying?' they asked him.

'Learning to juggle,' he said. That did not surprise me. In our group of friends, Simon had become renowned for his juggling skills. He could do it with erasers, cups, balls – anything, really.

His mother and father even tried asking me if I knew what had happened. I didn't want to say that Simon could only juggle if he was reasonably sober. As well as discovering juggling, he had discovered alcohol and often got quietly sozzled in his room. Sometimes we joined him around illicit bottles of cider – I don't know how he persuaded off-licences, much stricter in those days, to sell it to him. Mostly, we knew when to stop. And Simon just didn't. It was incredible he managed to keep this habit from his grandmother and his parents, but apparently he did.

And what had driven my friend to drink? Fiona. She was at the girls' grammar school and Simon had fallen hopelessly in love with her at a dance. Everyone had, but Simon was head over heels. She was recognized as the most beautiful girl in the area, and I daresay quite a lot of old men who once went to the boys' grammar still remember how, as she walked out of the school gates, she used to shake her head lazily and release her long blonde tresses to the wind.

Fiona did not return Simon's great and overwhelming love. She went out with him a few times but always in a group, and it seemed the more fawning his adoration, the more she simply scorned it. She preferred hunky rugby players. Simon was the clever, skinny type who kept bumping into things, partly because he removed his glasses when she was around.

Simon's parents were furious with the school at his A-level results. They demanded to know why no one had warned them that this might happen: they would have paid a tutor for extra help. They asked me if he had really been attending lessons. I said he had. And he had – in body. But, for a long time now, his soul had been absent.

For two years, I had been waiting for the Simon I knew to come back. Sometimes he was his old self, but less and less. We shared an interest in and enthusiasm for flight. In my case, this meant looking at aeroplanes from the ground and dreaming, my father being a devotee of what is now called the staycation. Simon, however, had been on many summer holidays abroad and I would ask him to tell me how it had felt when the plane took off and how it had felt when it landed. When it banked. When it cruised. When it did anything, really.

We lived under one flight path into Heathrow and we were plane watchers in a most desultory way: that is, we often looked up and tried to identify aircraft. Then, when we were seventeen, something amazing happened. The nation was enthralled by Concorde, the extraordinary V-shaped aeroplane that had been years in the making and which could fly faster than the speed of sound. Now it was scheduled to fly over central London with the Red Arrows. I had discovered the route. And it included Watford!

I had a Saturday job there (selling carpets at John Lewis, since you ask), but that day I was waiting on the shop roof for Concorde. I didn't care if I was sacked for this; nothing seemed more important. We had pored over maps and timings together, and Simon would also be watching from his house, I was sure of that.

I do not think I will ever forget the moment when Concorde — vast, white, dazzling, flanked by the tiny Red Arrows in razor-sharp formation — cut through a gin-clear sky over my right shoulder and turned towards central London. The sheer perfection of it. Glorious. The sort of perfection that could bring a tear to the eye. I watched the aeroplanes go, getting smaller and smaller with great rapidity until the Red Arrows had disappeared completely and even Concorde was a tiny dot. I kept staring at the sky they had left behind. Had they really been there? Had I really seen that? I knew it would take at least a week for my excitement to abate. And I knew that I really had to get into an aeroplane soon.

On my way home, I stopped at Simon's house.

'Wasn't it amazing!' I cried, the minute he opened the door.

Simon had that flat, detached look he had adopted lately.

'What?' he asked.

I stared at him in disbelief.

'Oh yeah,' he said, shrugging. 'Concorde. I forgot to look.'

It was hard to believe that this was my mate Simon. His voice empty of emotion, a strange disinterest in the world. Where had it come from? Deep down, I wasn't astonished when he failed his A-levels. He had stopped caring.

Most of us didn't get the grades we aspired to. No doubt this was because we all spent far too much time mooning over girls or hunched over transistor radios in our bedrooms. I avoided disturbing our house's inviolable quiet by wearing an enormous set of headphones with a long, long lead. Radio Caroline. Radio Luxembourg. Kenny Everett.

Dave Cash. In our rooms, we listened as fugitives from the BBC, drinking in every word, every note and every advert. It was the late 1960s and we knew that culture was breaking because here was musical freedom! It was thrilling. Equations and chemical formulae sat abandoned on our desks.

As for relationships, there were of course no mobile phones and, in our house, as in many others, there was just a black Bakelite telephone with a brown, plaited lead on a shelf in the hallway. Impossible, once I had a girlfriend, to murmur sweet nothings to her in private all evening: after two minutes my father was there in the hallway, demanding to know who was paying for the call. I think I did bring her home to meet my slightly disapproving father and the ever-present but almost completely absent Joyce. But my girlfriend was part of my other life, the life outside. Simon had developed another life, too, but his was inside his parents' four walls — or, more accurately, inside his own head.

Only years later did it occur to me that Simon must have been seriously depressed. And also that I had wrongly blamed Fiona for everything when in fact she was not the cause but simply the trigger for the explosive charge already buried in Simon. At the time, 'adolescent depression' was not a widely used phrase or even a recognized diagnosis. We were still post-war in so many ways and a stiff upper lip was expected, even by his high-achieving parents. They felt he had let them down and, despite being very nice people, they could not help showing it.

Only now do I understand that depression must explain his vacancy during lessons, the secret drinking which had gone far beyond schoolboy experimentation and the way my confident friend had turned into someone who could barely engage at all with the world.

My own A-level results had proved less than brilliant and I did not meet the grades required by my conditional offer to study medicine. After a tense few days I was accepted through clearing by University College London. I hoped I wasn't filling the place that Simon had vacated. I was sad and sorry for him but also secretly relieved that I had not been the one to totally fail my A-levels. My father's reaction would have been, frankly, terrifying. I had certainly feared a Vesuvian response to my mediocre results but, instead, to my relief, he was very supportive as I negotiated my way through the clearing system.

And so I went off to University College to start my long medical training. Simon did eventually make it to UCL, but after that strange diversion into what was, at the very least, extreme unhappiness, and perhaps a mental-health crisis. He was never exactly the same. Something had caused him to lose his footing, emotionally and academically. When we stood at the student bar together, it took me a while to realize that he was with people at each end and had drinks lined up with both groups.

I found myself worrying about him. Finally, I went to a highly respected professor to share my concern about my friend. He nodded. Simon had arrived drunk and garrulous at one of this man's electrifying lectures, so he was aware of the problem.

'Don't worry,' the professor confided later. 'I've had a word with him and we've got things under control. I've promised him a bottle of whisky if he passes his exams.'

He was the professor, so I did not dare argue with his doubtful logic.

Something about the young man whose body lay before me now reminded me of Simon. I suspected that here was someone who had lost himself at this age. And was the girl in the tent perhaps another Fiona?

We retreated while Jay was tidied up and the room given a thorough forensic clean before Amelia was wheeled in from the viewing room. Her parents had arrived to identify her there while we were busy with Jay. We fell silent when her mother's sobs, as she left the building, could be heard echoing from far down the corridor. When a shift of mortuary staff came in for their break and a cup of tea, we went off to change into clean scrubs before returning to the post-mortem room.

Amelia looked painfully young and sweet. Having encountered pregnancies in girls younger than twelve in the past, I assumed, perhaps wrongly, that a sexual relationship between Amelia and Jay was very likely. We carefully took off her distinctly unsexual flannel pyjamas: they had teddy bears embroidered on them. The cold weather may have curtailed any sexual activity between the couple. Or, by packing these pyjamas, she had, perhaps, been signalling a low level of interest or anticipation.

Naked, she looked even younger: small-breasted, skinny-waisted, with very little body hair. Rigor mortis had already passed on her slim, childish frame but her body retained the pink colouring of a cheap doll, or a carbon monoxide victim. When I examined her, she was distinctly pink inside as well. There was no doubt that her blood saturation level of CO would be high – even the blood sample I took for toxicology was not the usual dull red but an unnatural Barbie pink.

To establish that she had no underlying problems, I carefully examined, as always, all the systems of her body and her internal organs. After taking a routine urine sample from her bladder, I looked at her uterus – otherwise, of course, known as the womb.

The DI leaned forward. He was hoping for a pregnancy, which he thought, I'm not sure how, would further support his theory about these two deaths.

The uterus is the steely brown of clams which cling to rocks at the seaside. It is much more compact than a clam – if I form a circle with my thumb and forefinger, it will fit snugly inside. But it does have the same markedly triangular shape. The analogy ends there because the uterus has nothing of a shell's hardness. It is, however, firm. Firmer than any leg muscle, even the leg muscle of a habitual runner.

The triangular shape is inverted in the body. The tip, pointing south, is the cervix. This is the neck of the womb and, if its owner has had children, it may be as long as three centimetres. It links the uterus with the vagina.

At first sight, the cavity inside the uterus looks like nothing more than a slit. This seems to be surrounded by walls of solid muscle but is actually lined by a layer of very specialized cells: the endometrium. These cells grow and thicken during the first part of the menstrual cycle, making a soft, succulent and sustaining bed which heaves with spiral arteries. Just in case a fertilized egg lands. If that doesn't happen, then hormone levels fall, the lining breaks down and menstruation occurs.

The muscle of the uterine wall has an obvious role in childbirth, but for the nine months before that it must both grow and relax. This allows the cavity to enlarge enough to accommodate a growing foetus and, finally, a three-kilo baby. How can a clam turn into a basketball so easily? And then, after birth, revert back to, if not exactly a clam, then certainly something the size of a tennis ball? That is just one of the many miracles of pregnancy.

Another miracle is that the mother actually allows the

invasion of a growing embryo – which is, after all, a foreign body. Under any other circumstances, if you simply implant tissue from another person, the body's immune system will attack and destroy it. That is why surgical organ transplantation is successful only with the help of complex immunosuppressant therapies. So I find it amazing that mothers do not reject embryos – although, sadly, there are exceptions.

At the top of the uterus, the Fallopian tubes wander towards the ovaries, not in a straight line but with the elegant curve of a violin. Curiously, these tubes don't actually connect to the ovaries. They end in tiny fingers just above and around the ovaries, so that they caress without touching them. The inner lining of the tubes and of these tiny fingers are covered with cilia, projections that scoop or, you could say, waft an egg which has been released by the ovaries into the Fallopian tubes. There's something a bit vague about all this wafting. It seems distinctly hit and miss. Most of the time, the system operates efficiently, but not always. Released eggs can and do fail to find the tube and may end up in the abdominal cavity, where they are, like unused sperm, reabsorbed and recycled.

If a sperm is really agile, or the egg a little late, the egg may become fertilized before it even enters the Fallopian tube. Most will simply continue their journey and get wafted to the welcoming wall of the uterus. Occasionally, one may lose its way, in which case the fertilized egg will usually just fade away in the abdomen. But very rarely, a fertilized egg can stimulate the lining of the abdomen, the peritoneum, the ovary or even the bowel, to produce enough blood vessels to keep it supplied with oxygen and food. The pregnancy therefore continues, but usually only for a short time, in what is an inhospitable place for the growing foetus and a potentially fatal place for the mother.

Another mishap, and a slightly more common one, is that the fertilized egg sets off down the Fallopian tube towards the uterus but gets stuck and begins to grow in the tube itself. Pregnancies growing outside the womb are called ectopic and they can rapidly become obstetric emergencies. Fortunately, they are now usually detected and dealt with very rapidly in developed countries. However, there are still many parts of the world where nature's design glitch can lead to a mother bleeding to death.

The ovaries sit east and west of the top of the uterus and, technically, they are situated just inside the abdominal cavity. The word 'cavity' might give the impression of a vast, empty, echoing chamber, but that is not true at all. The so-called cavity is more like an overstuffed suitcase, full of organs, muscles, nerves and blood vessels. And, of course, thirty feet of intestines have to go somewhere. Apart from six inches at the top and bottom, they go here. One significant disadvantage of the position of the ovaries inside this packed suitcase is that ovarian cancer, that silent killer of older women, can, unnoticed, grow and spread very easily throughout the cavity – giving the tumour fast access to many other sites in the body.

Just as ovaries store eggs, the testes store sperm. But the similarities between ovaries and testes end there. A woman cannot manufacture more eggs than she is born with, and they are a declining asset. A female foetus may have 6 to 7 million eggs, but by birth the baby girl may have only 1 million. By puberty, most of these have degenerated, leaving a quarter of a million. And they may have to wait forty years or more for release. All this, while the testes are busy manufacturing sperm continually throughout a man's long reproductive life.

Each egg that remains at puberty is stored inside a small package called a follicle within the ovary. Right up until menopause, fluctuating hormone levels will instruct just one follicle to ripen its egg approximately every twenty-eight days. When the egg is mature, the follicle ruptures. Released by the ovary, it is, we hope, wafted into the Fallopian tube.

The ovaries which house these precious eggs are a redder colour than the uterus and are about the size of walnuts. As a woman ages, their surfaces become more irregular. The monthly rupture of follicles tends to leave them pitted and scarred over time – something that was certainly not true of Amelia's smooth, rounded ovaries.

I did not think, looking at her uterus on the outside, that she was pregnant.

The detectives' faces fell.

'Well, it's not enlarged. And when a woman's pregnant her womb goes sort of soft. It becomes very vascular . . . but let's take a look inside,' I said.

I cut open the uterus. There was no foetus visible to the human eye. And the crack where it might have been did not have the thick, vascular lining of pregnancy.

'How pregnant would she have to be, for you to see something?' the DI demanded.

'Depends when you start the clock. Pathologically, we can possibly detect something at a few weeks . . . let's see if we can find any signs of where she was in her menstrual cycle.'

I looked at the ovaries. One was larger than the other and a bit lopsided. When I opened it, embedded like a huge pearl was a yellow orb. A corpus luteum. Its egg-yolk colour filled more than half of the section I had cut. It really is one of the body's most remarkable sights.

'Ah,' I said.

The officers all looked from Amelia to me.

Nineteen or so days ago, the corpus luteum would have been a dull follicle ready to rupture and release an egg. Soon after the egg had gone, it had puffed itself up and got dressed in vibrant gold. It was now, temporarily, a spectacular hormone gland. I find this colour in only one other place, the inner adrenal glands, which are another site of hormone production. The yellow comes from carotene in the diet, for instance from carrots, tomatoes or squashes.

In this case, no sperm had fertilized the egg after release. There was no need for the corpus luteum to play nurse by secreting hormones to help maintain the very early stages of pregnancy. It does this until the placenta is big enough to take over hormone production and nursing care. If there is no pregnancy, as here, the corpus luteum will slowly take off its colourful scrubs and degenerate into a small, grey, unemployed nursemaid. The womb sheds its lining, menstruation takes place and another cycle begins.

'I don't think she can have been pregnant,' I said. 'This showy yellow tells me that the last egg Amelia released wasn't fertilized and so she had probably just finished her last period and was starting on her next cycle.'

'But you're going to check whether they had sex before she died?' the DI asked.

'Yep, I've swabbed her vagina and the lab will tell us if there's semen present.'

I had given him no evidence to support his theory, but the examination seemed to make the DI sure of himself.

'Yeah,' he said decisively. 'It's got to be a murder-suicide.'

'That would be very unusual in this age group,' I told him. 'It's something that I associate with midlife.'

He failed to digest this.

'When did they die?' he demanded.

I did not have time to reply before he half answered his own question.

'I mean, she went first, obviously. But how long afterwards do you think he topped himself?'

As always, this was going to be tricky. It was Sunday night now, and the pair had seemingly died on Friday night. Medicine is not so exact that it is possible to pinpoint the exact time of either death at such a distance.

'I'll work on that,' I told him. And I did, later at home, with charts and formulae. But I could reach no satisfactory conclusion. All the pencil-chewing and head-scratching just confirmed what I already suspected: that they had both died between 9 p.m. Friday and 9 a.m. Saturday. That was as accurate as I could be.

When the blood tests came back, they showed that Amelia's blood saturation of CO was 58 per cent. It was not surprising that she had died of carbon monoxide poisoning and it seemed obvious to me that this was caused by bringing the barbecue – probably still warm and covertly smouldering – into the tent.

Of course, no one could ever know for certain if Jay, according to the police theory, had been told the relationship was over and had then decided to deliberately arrange Amelia's death. But the police awaited his blood saturation results keenly: the lower his CO saturation, the more they believed their theory was vindicated. What they really wanted was a level of zero, indicating that he must have left Amelia alone with the barbecue and barely even entered the tent himself.

Jay's results arrived the next day and showed a carbon

monoxide level of 29 per cent. I had to admit that, in two similarly young and fit people subjected to the same exposure at the same time, this was a large difference. But Jay had been in the open air at the cliff after exposure and Amelia had remained in the tent and died. So it needed explanation, but it was not astonishing.

I did not personally give much credence to the police theory that Amelia's death was a homicide. Of course, seventeen-year-old boys do kill, and most certainly they are killed, but this is usually in a fit of uncontrolled fury or passion, or it is required by the brotherhood in gang warfare. I simply could not imagine a teenager murdering a girlfriend in such an unusual, planned, cold-blooded way. It seemed much more likely that the pair had not known that the cooling barbecue was lethal than that one of them had used it as a murder weapon.

Some interesting forensic evidence emerged a little later to show that the cigarette butts found at the top of the cliff had not all been smoked by Jay. Amelia's DNA was also found on them. In fact, toxicology confirmed the presence of both nicotine and cannabis in a couple of the butts and in both Jay and Amelia.

I suspected that the couple had discovered the place at the top of the cliff much earlier and had smoked a few joints there. I thought that at night they had innocently taken their barbecue into the tent for warmth. I believed that Jay had woken with, probably, a pounding headache, nausea and confusion. He left the tent to be sick. He may have thought it was the food they had eaten or maybe the cannabis they had smoked. I doubt he realized Amelia was dead; more likely, he assumed that she was well and asleep. Either way, he somehow found his way back to the clifftop in the dark, in a confused mental state. Once there, he may have jumped. Or he had simply fallen over the edge, and of the two possibilities I thought this was more probable.

Teenagers will always have a propensity to explore, to stride further and more defiantly from the parental wing than ever before, to question the rules, beliefs and authority of the family, to wrongly assume that strangers will be as cherishing – or as uncaring – as home. And they are often determined to experiment with anything parents have warned against. Teenage deaths, though few, reflect this need to explore and become independent. Statistically, accidents and suicide are far more likely than other deaths in this age group. In fact, suicide is now a leading cause of death for under-twenty-fives. Numbers have increased inexorably in both sexes, but there are still many more male suicides than female. However, since 2012, the incidence in young women has almost doubled.

A theory based entirely on statistics, therefore, might suggest that Amelia had shoved Jay down the cliff when he was slightly incapacitated by marijuana and had then gone back to the tent to gas herself. Nobody even suggested that scenario, but there was just as much evidence for it as for the police's murder-suicide hypothesis. All we can learn from this is that no sensible theory was ever extracted from mortality statistics. Each case is unique.

At the inquest, the coroner heard from me, the police and from the two teenagers' devastated families. He said he did not have enough evidence to record a verdict of suicide for Jay: it simply was not clear if the boy had jumped or fallen or even been pushed. He recorded an open verdict.

The coroner also had to decide whether there was a possibility that Jay had deliberately killed Amelia with the barbecue.

Or if she had killed herself. Or whether her death was an accident. Probably Jay's parents were hoping Amelia's verdict would be accidental death, thus ending newspaper speculation about their son's culpability. As I sat in court, I recalled that he was their only child. I tried not to flinch from their sheet-white, hollow-eyed faces. Nor from Amelia's traumatized parents, who held on to each other as I gave evidence. At the end of the inquest, they were all to be disappointed. The coroner recorded, on Amelia's death, too, an open verdict.

An open verdict may not bring families the closure they crave, and it may not shut the door to endless speculation, but it does firmly put on record an unpalatable fact: that sometimes we will never be able to know with certainty exactly what happened.

Then a soldier,
Full of strange oaths, and bearded like the pard,
Jealous in honour, sudden and quick in quarrel,
Seeking the bubble reputation
Even in the cannon's mouth.

7

One of the police officers formally identified the young man who lay in the post-mortem room as Andrew Styler. Another gave Andrew's age as twenty-four.

'What job did he do?' I asked the officers.

I usually have the chance to ask this kind of question before a post-mortem. The police brief me in the staff tea-room, where the tea is hot, or the relative comfort of the bereavement room if there are no grieving families around. Here we can watch the fish circle in their tank while we nurse cups of cool tea and eat broken biscuits.

Today, however, the officers had been late and anxious to start immediately. We had changed and gone straight into the post-mortem room, and I knew only one thing about the deceased: he had fallen off a wall and hit his head.

He lay before us, face up. He was well-shaven and had the haircut of a man who cares about his appearance. His forehead and cheeks had been noticeably grazed on one side. I surveyed him closely as the photographer manoeuvred into position. For a strange, dazzling second, light bounced off the walls, the metal surfaces, the body and even off our faces.

'Head next?'

He had just photographed the whole body and was an old hand. It was obvious to him that the cause of death was a head injury. As well as the facial grazing, there was blood visible on the neck and more blood had clearly been leaking from one of Andrew's ears into his dark hair.

I said: 'Let's have a good look at him first.'

Careful study of the body's exterior can be as revealing as anything found inside it. Yes, there was certainly a head injury here, but we'd get to that. If you think you know the cause of death and go straight to it, you might so easily miss something else that is relevant. It is essential to take a really good look at the rest of the body, starting as far away from the suspected cause of death as possible. So, of course, I began at Andrew's feet. After examining them carefully, my focus moved slowly north, searching for bruises, abrasions, perhaps signs of a fight or a scuffle: any information that might tell me his story.

His hands were grazed, probably where he'd tried to break his fall and save his head. There were no other apparent injuries. But instinct and experience told me something wasn't right about him. What, though?

I turned him over. His shoulders were bruised: he'd evidently fallen headfirst and landed on a hard surface and then bounced. Despite the grazing to his face, it was clear that he'd fallen backwards – at the back of his head were swelling, slight bleeding and evident abrasion.

I kept casting an eye down his body and my eye kept resting on his legs. They looked normal enough at a glance but, when I stared hard at them, I could see that each one was different.

By now the coroner's officer had finished flicking through her notes and could answer my question.

'Apparently he did something in the City. Worked for Wagners, it says. What do they do?'

'Insurance,' one of the detectives said.

I turned Andrew over again, the photographer backed off and everyone moved closer. I noticed his hair again. His quiff must have flopped annoyingly over his eyes when he was alive.

'So what do we know about him?' I asked.

'Er . . . recently married, got a baby at home, but he went out last night with his mates . . .'

'Ah, mates,' I said. Mates can turn nasty with each other surprisingly rapidly, even, under certain circumstances, very close mates.

'And his brother,' the young detective constable added.

'Ah, brothers,' I said. Brothers, too, can turn nasty.

'They both have the same mates. There's only a year between them,' the inspector said.

'It was the brother who pushed him,' the detective constable explained helpfully.

There was a silence. The inspector looked at him hard and then swallowed.

'Allegedly,' he said.

I hate receiving these stories piecemeal. It would have been so much more productive to have sat down with a cup of tea beforehand, learned all about the case and asked lots of questions then.

'So, do we know what actually happened?'

The detective sergeant took over. 'Well, apparently, these two come from a very competitive family. Both good at sport, but the younger brother's just getting to the stage where he's outshining Andrew, and he's not going to let his big brother forget it. A lot of teasing because Andrew's been dropped from the football team they both play for. And then some stuff about how Andrew's been a waste of space ever since he became a father. No one hears what Andrew says to that but, whatever it is, the brother gets very angry. He says . . .'

The sergeant paused so long that the inspector reached for his own notes and read the quote himself. His delivery was leaden. He wasn't much of an actor: '"I'd like to kill you. I've always wanted to kill you."'

Never say that. Especially not if you're planning to kill someone. But even if you aren't, those words could mean you face a lot of awkward questions one day.

The sergeant carried on. 'Seems the little brother has recently taken up parkour . . .'

As if a button had been pressed, everyone in the room groaned. Everyone except Andrew, of course, and me.

'Did you say parking?' I asked.

'Parkour. It's a sport, sort of. A few girls, but mostly lads. They start running and they don't stop, no matter what's in their way. They don't like to run around things. So they go over, along, up, down . . .'

'I'd give it a go if I was twenty years younger and ten times fitter,' the coroner's officer said. 'I mean, you don't see them pause to think about it. Looks spectacular.'

'Yeah, until they die.'

I was still examining Andrew, but now I looked up. I'd never heard of this.

'They climb walls, trees – anything. They walk along high ledges, leap from pillar to pillar, vault over fences . . .'

'They'll go up on to the top of one tall building in Regent Street and then jump from roof to roof and, before you know it, they're in Green Park. I bet some of them make a fortune on YouTube with the footage.'

I asked: 'Is it a sort of race?'

They shook their heads. 'More like a martial art. The serious ones do a lot of training.'

'They're the ones who don't hurt themselves?'

'Except sometimes they do,' the boss said. 'I mean, they're super-fit, but they can make mistakes.'

'It's the amateurs who're worse,' the coroner's officer said. 'They have a few pints and think they can do parkour, too.'

I made an incision over the top of Andrew's right thigh to take blood from his femoral vein to send to toxicology. They would soon tell us what drugs or alcohol he might have consumed before death. Blood alcohol levels are a factor in many, many deaths – and, in the case of homicide, that can be as true of the victim as the perpetrator.

'What do they wear? These parkour people?' I asked.

The paramedics had cut most of Andrew's clothes in their attempts to resuscitate but, when he'd been wheeled in, he'd been wearing what was left of a business suit.

'Athletic stuff,' they all agreed. 'Not suits.'

'So you're telling me that a man who worked in insurance had a few drinks with a bunch of mates, including his brother, and they all decided to try this parkour . . .'

The detective sergeant nodded. 'Yeah, the younger brother's started parkour training and I daresay he wants to show off a bit. Trying to make his big brother look small.'

'Yeah, a lot of teasing going on, and apparently it did get a bit nasty,' the inspector added.

'And they were walking along a wall –'

'Running.'

'How high was it?'

'Six feet, maybe, not even that.'

'They took steps up to a shop roof then jumped down on to a garage roof and then down further on to this wall. Not difficult stuff by parkour standards. And now they're running along the wall. Gardens on one side, hard pavement on the other.'

'And you're saying the younger brother pushes Andrew off the wall?'

'According to no less than three witnesses.'

I wasn't sure that the statements of a group of drunken lads would carry much weight in court.

'And,' the inspector said, 'there was a lady watching them from her bedroom window; it was her neighbour's wall they were on. And she's sure she saw the one behind give the one in front a shove.'

The sergeant said: 'The brother doesn't deny that he touched Andrew. But he says' – and here his tone was derisory – 'he says he was trying to steady him.'

The young detective constable had made up his mind.

'Yeah. Right.' His voice was heavy with cynicism.

I said: 'So you're after the brother for manslaughter?'

'Or,' the inspector said, 'perhaps worse.'

Murder seemed a harsh charge in the circumstances. I found myself feeling sorry for the younger brother. He might have unkindly put a hand on Andrew, intending him to fall a few feet to the ground. But that's very different from trying to kill him by pushing him head down on to hard paving.

'How is the brother now?' I asked.

The detective constable said: 'Distraught.'

'Remorseful?' the inspector asked sharply.

'He's not there yet, because he's still saying he didn't do anything wrong.'

I said: 'If Andrew had been drinking, then he wouldn't have been steady on his feet. You could have trouble pressing charges.'

The inspector shook his head: 'Actually, we think he was sober. According to all the lads, Andrew cut back on his drinking once he became a family man. So, of course, he gets teased about that, too, by his kid brother.'

At least in Andrew's case we knew what the row was about. Often, the cause of a fatal dispute is a fact which barely sees the light of day: life's illogical arguments, petty resentments, small justifications – well, they all just evaporate in the face of death's enormity.

I warned them: 'I may disappoint you if you're hoping I can tell you whether Andrew fell or was pushed. Not unless he was pushed so harshly that there are bruises to prove it, or unless I can find gripping injuries.'

But I already knew that there were no unexplained bruises and no gripping injuries. Sometimes these emerge a few days after death so, expecting little, I made a note to myself to meet Andrew again in a day or two. Even as I began to open him up, I didn't expect to find much information internally that would shed light on whether he had fallen or been pushed. Push/fall is at the heart of the homicide/accident interface, and that interface is a very tricky and sensitive place. Pathology plays a vital role, but it is part of a wider picture that includes the whole history of the case, the circumstances, an analysis of the relevant relationships, plus any witness statements. Even with all this information, there is often insufficient evidence to prosecute.

I cut down the midline and folded back the skin and fat. Almost everyone in Western society has fat clinging to the underside of their skin, even a fit young man. Now the two pectoralis major muscles, one on either side of the chest, bulged at me. At first sight these muscles are, like almost everything else in the body, surrounded by a spider's web of connective tissue but, when I swiped this gently aside with a finger, it collapsed like pulled cotton wool and all but disappeared. The muscle beneath was a healthy red-brown. In fact, at twenty-four, Andrew's body looked as good as it gets.

The pecs are shaped like a hand. Its wrist joins the upper part of the humerus (the bone of the upper arm) and, like a thumb, a little separate part tags on to the bottom of the inner clavicle. The pectoral 'fingers' are tight together and fan out across the chest to the sternum – that's the bone running down the centre of the ribs. This span makes the pectoralis major a long muscle – maybe ten to fifteen centimetres – and in Andrew's case, at about 1.5 cm, it was also quite thick. The pecs are essential for many arm movements, but, and often more importantly, they can also dramatically change the contour of the upper chest. So some people, particularly young men, regard the development of these muscles as important. I would say, looking at the thickness and curvature here, that Andrew had either spent long hours weightlifting in the gym or, much less likely, he had taken anabolic steroids. So, did all that effort make his muscle rock-hard? Did those weeks, months or even years of training mean my trusty PM40 scalpel had difficulty cutting through his pectoralis major? Not at all. It took no extra time and required no extra effort. Who wants to be the fittest corpse in the mortuary anyway?

The meat we eat is animal muscle and it is little different in appearance to the muscle inside our own bodies. First-timers in the post-mortem room are sometimes shocked to find that steak is the word which leaps to mind. It is possible to see tiny fibres in the muscles with the naked eye, all running in the same direction. Under a microscope these fibres are revealed as bundles and inside the bundles are more bundles, and inside them – and we really are at a microscopic level now – nestle still more bundles. These enable a muscle to do absolutely the only thing a muscle can do. Contract. That is, they get shorter. Nothing else. Muscles are a one-trick wonder.

The instruction to contract comes from the brain, of course – throw that ball! – and is relayed through the nerves. Just like the veins and arteries that accompany them, nerves become increasingly smaller and more branched as they become more peripheral, eventually reaching and spreading over their destination muscle. Nerve is connected to muscle by tiny buttons. They remind me of the rectangular PP3 batteries of my boyhood, which had cups and clasps, how they clipped so neatly and reciprocally into place. Once the instruction to throw that ball is received at these muscle buttons, dramatic changes in calcium concentration prompt the chemical and electrical process which enables a muscle to do what it is designed for. It contracts. And suddenly the ball is in the air.

Muscles appear boring, because their surface appearance is uniform in texture and colour. Muscles are actually fascinating, because they come in all shapes and sizes and are joined to bones in many different ways, depending on their function. This means that our bodies can flex, stretch, rotate and contort extraordinarily – without our muscles performing more than their one simple trick. Contraction.

For the pathologist, although there are often good reasons to examine muscles, it's usually a question of moving them out of the way to reach more interesting parts of the body. They form a thick but predictable patchwork blanket over the cavities, organs and bones that can reveal so many secrets. I couldn't even begin to examine Andrew for rib fractures without moving the pectoralis major muscles, both of them, and their buddies, the pectoralis minor muscles, that lie underneath and move the shoulder blades.

There were no rib fractures and no bruises, so I turned towards the most obvious injury and was not surprised to find a fractured skull and, in the brain, bleeding.

Beneath the skull are three layers of membrane which get thinner the nearer the brain, so that the thinnest of all wraps itself tightly to the surface of the brain and is almost invisible to the naked eye. It is separated by little more than a slimy film from the middle membrane, the arachnoid layer. This delicate, translucent sheet is easy to see through, and no special skills are required to pick it up with the forceps and pull it out of the way. Above it, cushioned by special fluid produced deep within the brain – the cerebrospinal fluid – and tethered to the arachnoid layer by tiny veins, is the dura.

Most haemorrhages inside the skull are caused by trauma, but some just happen of their own accord. A haemorrhage just under the arachnoid layer, for instance, is most commonly caused by a punch or a kick, but it can also happen out of the blue to an apparently healthy young person who is doing something as innocuous as loading the dishwasher. Of course, there is a reason for this, and it's another case of foul play by genes. The patient generally has no idea that they were born with a weakness in the walls of one or more arteries inside their skull. There is a roundabout of arteries at the base of the brain called the Circle of Willis and here the artery walls are prone to congenital weakness. A small bubble may develop in this area which, when it bursts, causes a subarachnoid haemorrhage, resulting in misery and sometimes immediate death. But some such bubbles never burst. I have found them – they are called berry aneurysms because they look like small berries – in the bodies of old people who have died for unrelated reasons, so they are not always fatal and may be completely symptomless.

I should say that the Circle of Willis tends to have rather more corners than you might expect of a circle. And to understand why its complex knot of vessels is such a weak point for aneurysms, just think of the early jet passenger planes. No one could understand why the previously safe Comets suddenly started to crash in the 1950s. They had square windows – houses have square windows, why wouldn't aeroplanes? – and eventually, when the aircraft had clocked up enough hours for stresses to show, the sharp corners of the windows were found to be an area of great weakness. The result was cracks in the fuselage. And that is why aircraft have curved windows. Unfortunately, though, there is no chance of redesigning the human body with fewer sharp corners.

Andrew had died from a haemorrhage, but his was a different type of bleeding. It was between the arachnoid layer and the dural layer. Subdural haemorrhages are almost always caused by trauma.

The dura lies directly under the skull, so close to the bone that it is practically stuck to it; prising it away from the inner surface of the skull can take a lot of time and effort and may cause pathologists to swear. This dura is off-white and as tough as strong canvas, although it does not quite have the thickness of a Boy Scout tent. And it has no give at all. When it finally comes away from the skull, there may be a distinctive ripping sound.

Andrew had died almost at once and blood, therefore, had little time to escape from the small, dense veins which pack the space beneath the dura and were now torn away. His haemorrhage was perhaps a centimetre thick and extended over the surface of the brain for five centimetres or so. There is a doubtful medical habit, started in the seventeenth century, of describing the body, diseases and abnormalities, in culinary terms. At the risk of perpetuating this dubious tradition, I would say that a subdural haemorrhage most resembles a large blob of redcurrant jelly.

However, the bleeding from the tiny, torn subdural veins over the surface of the brain had not killed Andrew. He had died of trauma to the cerebral tissue itself. In events far too quick for the human eye, slow-motion replays of falls show us that when someone lands on their head it distorts and rotates before bouncing. Onlookers see and remember that bounce. But they tend to miss the crucial part – because it is the distortion and rotation that are the killers.

The brain is divided into many discrete areas and each has a different tolerance and resilience to trauma. Scoops of ice cream in a cone, each with its own flavour and consistency, will separate if the cone is shaken hard enough, and that is what can happen to the traumatized brain: the different structures, some more robust than others, move in different directions in different ways and at different speeds. The axons of nerves passing through or between these areas are ripped apart. And the likelihood of tearing is greatly worsened by the micro-seconds of rotation.

Once injured, brain tissue, like all injured tissues, will swell. But the skull is, of course, completely inelastic. Bounded by this solid box, the expanding brain has nowhere to go and, if the injury is to one side, as that side of the brain swells it may even push itself right across the skull's midline in an attempt to find more space.

Andrew's haemorrhage was obvious to the naked eye, but the shearing and tearing were not. Beyond the blob of the subdural haemorrhage, and apart from other small bleeds around the fracture itself, his brain looked perfect. As I held it in my hands, firm and, indeed, beautiful, I marvelled, as always, at this amazing anatomical phenomenon.

From early adulthood until it starts to atrophy in later life, the brain's appearance changes little. A lattice of small blood vessels overlays the outermost layer of the cortical ribbon. They follow the brain's extraordinary geography like mule tracks twisting around Alpine valleys seen from the air. Fly lower, and you can see how each has its own extensive network of tiny capillaries. It is possible to study these and find, as well as a rational vascular system, great art. I mean the art of a Van Gogh, with its sense of something organic and emotional outgrowing and overtaking the simply functional.

The way the arteries feed the brain with blood and the veins drain it away once its passage is complete is unique to this organ. The intricate beauty of the small vessels which give the brain its magnificent exterior hints at the extraordinary range of processes that flourish within: voluntary and involuntary actions, rational and irrational thought, the ability to learn, the ability to recall, to create and to do so much more. No organ has more complexity or mystery, within and without. None has more possibility of good or evil, none more beauty. Within and without.

We remove and weigh all the body's organs at post-mortem to help establish their normality, and the brain is no exception. For its size, it is quite weighty in the healthy young – similar to a bag of sugar. It feels like nothing else I know. After a bomb blast, when flesh and offal are scattered everywhere, it is possible to pick up some scattered tissue and know at once, from its consistency and colour, that here is an adult brain. Such recognition sears into your own brain. The feeling which follows can best be described as empathy in its most acute form.

It is easy enough to damage a brain with poor handling. But the brain is not so delicate that it loses its shape when free of the skull. I see it as a wonderful gift, the dura its wrapping and the skull the box in which it is safely sent. But even without the box and wrapping, the brain has sufficient density to maintain its form.

When I lifted Andrew's brain up for weighing, I felt its unique combination of softness and firmness. Can I compare it to a thick, set yoghurt? No, it's not sloppy at all. To jelly? Absolutely not; it does not wobble. To rice pudding? Not really; it retains its shape even if you pick it up and put it down and flip it over. To a soft cheese? Perhaps. Or maybe it might just be what it is, unique and simply defying comparison.

You might assume that, because Andrew had fallen initially on to the back of his head, that is where there was the most damage. In fact, the impact had passed through the bone at the top and the sides and then reunited, causing a fracture at the base of his skull. It took some time to examine and photograph all this and, when I had finished, I could sense the police officers were nearly ready to go home, to the pub, to be anywhere but here in the post-mortem room.

'So, in the end, you still can't tell if he was pushed or not?' The inspector sighed wearily.

But I knew that this wasn't the end and that we still had a long way to go. I looked at Andrew's legs again. It was time to address the feeling I'd had from the beginning. No beer, no TV, no tea. Not yet, anyway.

8

'Did you say he played a lot of football?' I asked.

The inspector looked impatient.

'What's that got to do with his head injury, Doc?'

I didn't answer. I wasn't sure.

The sergeant said: 'He used to play football at the weekend. But last night the brother, apparently quite nastily, told everyone he'd been dropped from the team. Andrew said that he'd decided to opt out because he'd rather be at home with the baby. And the brother called him . . .' He studied his notebook. '". . . a total wuss".'

'Did the brother say why he was dropped?' I asked.

'Now then, this is what really sparked the row.' There was a long pause while the sergeant scanned his pages. Finally, he found the right place. 'Ah, yes. So, the brother rubbished Andrew's recent football skills. Kept saying that he'd lost it and fell over the ball whenever it came near him.'

'Does anyone here play football?' I asked.

There was a silence. Finally the constable spoke up.

'I used to play a lot until I switched to squash.'

'What did it do to your legs?'

The constable stared at me.

'Nothing, really.'

'Did you have very strong calves?'

He looked thoughtful.

'My mum used to say you'd think I was a rugby player from my thighs. Can't remember much about my calves.'

By now everyone was staring at Andrew's legs.

'Anyone notice anything?' I asked.

'The left's bigger than the right,' the coroner's officer said at last.

'Only below the knee,' the sergeant said. 'Actually, now I really look, it's weird.'

'That calf's massive!' the constable agreed.

'Just big,' corrected the inspector.

I wrapped the measuring tape around each one in turn.

'Both calves are big, it's just the left's bigger.'

The inspector glanced at the clock.

'But what's it got to do with his head injury?' he asked again.

'I'm not sure,' I admitted.

I had my suspicions about that left leg; about the right, too. An enlarged calf can point to a deep vein thrombosis and I had to check for this first. A DVT would be an unusual find in a fit young man because a blood clot in the leg, although it can be caused by various factors, is most often the result of slow blood flow. This frequently follows a long period of inactivity – for instance after an operation. I wondered if Andrew spent hours sitting without moving in front of his computer at work.

'I wear these tight sock things when I fly to America to visit my daughter,' the coroner's officer said. 'So I don't get a DVT.' I guessed that she had seen enough blood clots at post-mortem over the years to learn some lessons.

'They're certainly a danger if you fly long haul and sit too still,' I said. 'Especially cramped in cattle class. Maybe Andrew had a holiday recently? Or a business trip?'

'Nothing in my notes about any travel,' the detective sergeant reported. 'But I can ask the family?'

'Not yet,' I told him.

DVT is very hazardous because the blood clot can break loose and travel up through the vein to the lungs, where it may be a rapid killer. If this had happened in Andrew's case, I would already have discovered it. But I still had to rule out DVT before I studied his legs further. I have seen it many times – and perhaps not seen it when I should have done. If there's no apparent reason to dissect the legs to look at the veins at post-mortem, we don't. So DVT, which is certainly not always visible at a glance, may often be missed by pathologists.

Instead of heading to the pub, the officers now waited patiently while I examined Andrew's left leg. In order to reach the vein, I had to cut through the complex muscles of the calf. These move the feet and are crucial for balance. I was very interested in these muscles but I had to double-check the vein first.

A blood clot, long and dark red, matches the shape of the vein but bulges from inside it, as if a snake has swallowed a broomstick. It didn't take long to establish that Andrew had no blood clots.

So now it was back to that muscle. I had known as soon as I touched it that something was wrong. I'm often asked how I can work and chat at the same time without looking at what I'm doing – and the answer is that my hands and fingers are constantly busy. They are feeling, touching, sensing. So much of pathology is about touch, and alarm bells ring when things aren't right. They were ringing now. Where I'd expected uniformity of texture, Andrew's muscle was uneven. In some places, the tissue was firm, fatty, fibrous – but not in others. I quickly examined the right leg. It was similar, but the muscle was perhaps not quite so pale and mottled, and it was a bit less fatty.

At last I looked up.

'Right,' I said. They all stared at me. 'Something very interesting is going on with these muscles, I'm not yet sure what.'

'So, have you finished?' Those pints were calling.

'I'm going to take a few samples of the muscle for microscopy. But it seems to me that a lot hinges on Andrew's blood alcohol level. If he had been drinking, even if he wasn't technically drunk, then you've really got no case against the brother. Andrew's a drunk larking about on a wall who wobbles and falls off.' I thought of my friend Simon's laughing face. No one could hide his drinking as well as Simon if he wanted to.

'Yeah,' the inspector said gloomily.

The keen detective constable said: 'But we've got all the witnesses!'

The sergeant shook his head. 'If Andrew was drunk, then the CPS won't listen to any number of witnesses who say he was pushed.'

'No, they'll say that he was simply asking for trouble, running on a wall when he's had a few,' I agreed.

Note to murderers: you might be more likely to get away with a push, shove or fall if your victim is drunk. I have noticed this many times over the years. Although you can't count on it.

'We'd better wait for the tox to tell us what his blood alcohol level was,' the inspector said, 'before we do anything else.'

He turned to the CSI. 'Let's put that through as urgent.'

But I did do something else. If my suspicions were correct, I felt morally impelled to act for the sake of Andrew's family. As well as submitting samples to establish his alcohol level, I took a few more blood samples for specialist tests.

We left the post-mortem room and got on with our lives

while we waited for the results, but I found myself preoccupied with the case. By the mid-twenties the brain is fully developed, and around this time young people often decide what they really want to do in life, or at least focus on what lies ahead.

My friend Simon had became quite serious at this stage. He had engaged with medicine at last and decided he really wanted to become an anaesthetist, he had a girlfriend who was a lot nicer than Fiona, and his career was progressing well. Whatever crisis had overtaken him in his late teens seemed far behind him now. He would still drink quite phenomenal amounts but, when sober, he was my funny, interesting, interested mate again.

Andrew had evidently changed at this age, too. He was no longer the drinker his brother remembered but had died at the beginning of an apparent period of stability in his life: a wife, a baby, a job in the City.

And what of his contemporaries who lack that stability? Latest figures show the suicide rate rising still further in those aged between twenty and thirty-four, accounting for more than 28 per cent of all male deaths and about 18 per cent of female deaths at this age. The next most likely cause is accidental poisoning, a catch-all phrase which might include being given the wrong prescription but generally means an unintended drugs overdose. Then car accidents, followed by homicide – because Shakespeare was right about young men being *jealous in honour, sudden and quick in quarrel,* particularly when under the influence of drugs or alcohol, which leads us to the fifth most common cause of death in the twenty- to thirty-four-year-old male: cirrhosis of the liver.

The statistics for young women are similar, but there is one major difference: breast cancer is already their third-biggest killer. Not far behind are car crashes and cirrhosis;

this last has shown a significant increase in this female cohort in the twenty-first century.

What do these statistics tell us about early adulthood? As we leave childhood behind, we take control of our lives and so become increasingly responsible for our own deaths. No one chooses to have cancer, of course, but fighting, driving dangerously and drinking or drug-taking to excess are at least theoretically under our control and therefore preventable – if the young choose to exercise this control. We are all familiar with youthful assumptions of immortality.

The first of Andrew's results to come back was from the specialist test I had requested: a creatine kinase test. This enzyme is found in healthy muscle cells but, if it is also present in the blood in significant amounts, then leakage has occurred – and leakage points to damage in the muscle cells. In Andrew's case, the raised enzyme level was evidence that the muscle damage was considerable, but I could not yet identify what form that damage took. My suspicion was that something had started to go wrong in the metabolic processes in the leg muscles, so we were still a long way from even beginning to make a diagnosis.

Andrew's blood alcohol level eventually arrived. It was just below 50 mg/100 ml, which put him well within the driving limit in England and right on the upper limit for driving in Scotland. His friends had been correct: he had not been drunk on the evening of his death. His brother was now a step closer to the dock.

As soon as the tox came through, I contacted the coroner's office to say I wanted to pursue my theory about Andrew's leg muscles. In fact, I had already been quietly and unofficially doing this: I'd looked at the formalin-fixed, laboratory-processed samples under a microscope, using all of the chemical stains available. I enjoyed the kaleidoscope of colours they made, but I was still struggling to understand the story. I reached for the phone.

'The police are likely pressing charges against the brother,' the coroner's officer said. 'And so there's no way the coroner's going to pay for some expensive expert to look down his microscope for you. Not when the CPS could be picking up the bill later.'

'I really believe this could be important evidence,' I insisted.

'The coroner's got a budget, you know.'

'Can I speak to him?'

'He's very busy today.'

'Can I phone him tomorrow?'

'I'll put you on his call list,' she said firmly. 'I'm sure he'll speak to you when he can.'

This coroner had been appointed recently. Over the years, I had become good mates with his predecessor, who would have rung me back at once.

'I've got a budget, you know,' said the new coroner when he finally made contact. 'And the rules for payment regarding microscopic studies are quite clear. I can't pay you any more. And anyway, the investigation of this murder is now solely in the hands of the police.'

Clearly, he was one of the new legal coroners. He knew everything about coronial law but not a lot about medicine, let alone how we establish crucial facts.

I said: 'I know that they're thinking of prosecuting the brother, but –'

'Exactly. So when they've charged him, you should talk to the police or the CPS if you think you've got some expensive evidence you want them to have.'

'This young man fell off a wall. Either it was an accident or he was pushed by his brother.'

'That's exactly what the police think, and it's what the witnesses are saying.'

I heard the sound of the finance door slamming shut in my face. But I persevered.

'I now believe there is a third possibility. I think there might have been a muscle disorder in the deceased's legs, but I need an expert to take a look.'

'If there was something that wrong, why didn't he go to a doctor?'

'He may not have known. He may not have wanted to know. What young person wants to admit he's falling over at soccer because he can't control his legs? I daresay he felt well otherwise.'

There was a long pause. The pause of a coroner doing maths.

'And it will cost £600 or so for this expert, you say?'

'About that, yes.'

'Then if the police won't stump up, I really think you'd better try the CPS, don't you?'

There was no doubt that this was the coroner's call, and I was sure his predecessor would have agreed to foot the bill. But I didn't want to get into a legal argument and, after a lot of to-ing and fro-ing, I persuaded the police to pay for a learned professor to review my slides with his electron microscope.

He soon phoned me.

'I'll submit a full report,' he said, 'but, basically, your lad had muscular dystrophy.'

Muscular dystrophy. Bad news for any family.

'Which one?' I asked, for this cruel condition is a many-headed snake.

'Becker's. Surprising it wasn't more obvious by the age of twenty-four, but I suspect that if you talked to family members, you'd probably find he's been a bit unsteady for a while.'

'He'd just been dropped from the football team,' I said.

'Quite an achievement to have stayed in it as long as he did, frankly.'

'What about the genetic implications here?'

'With Becker's MD, the mother's probably the carrier. Has he got any brothers?'

'Yes. In fact, the brother may be charged with his murder. They were running along a wall and witnesses said he pushed Andrew off it.'

The expert made a long, loud, honking noise of complete disbelief.

'What was he doing prancing on a wall when he had Becker's muscular dystrophy?'

'Will you say that in your report?'

'I'll say it was amazing he managed to clamber up there at all.'

'The brother will want testing for Becker's, too,' I said.

'Certainly will.'

'And the deceased became a father recently.'

'Well,' the expert said. 'If the baby's a girl, then she'll be a carrier. But he can't pass it on to a son.'

Becker's muscular dystrophy doesn't always show as early as some of the other MDs and people can live with it into their forties and often beyond, though they will become less and less active. The cause? Another unlucky number in the genetic lottery. This mutation occurs on one of the largest known human genes, the DMD gene, which is responsible for making dystrophin. This protein is one of many that are vital for maintaining healthy and sound muscles. It is largely absent in people with Becker's MD and, as the muscle is used over time, it becomes increasingly damaged until it finally weakens and dies. Andrew's calf muscles were the first to show the changes but, if he had lived, others would have followed. Unfortunately, in many cases of muscular dystrophy, the heart muscle is eventually affected.

Becker's MD is usually passed on via the X chromosome (of which women have two and men just one) from mother to son. Daughters can carry the gene and have a 50 per cent chance of passing it on to each son, but they are unlikely to show symptoms themselves: they have that second X chromosome to help with the dystrophin shortage. Andrew's brother, who had teased him so brutally about his loss of leg control, might soon start to experience the same loss himself. Specialist advice and counselling would be needed for the family. They had lost one son. Now they would want to know if they might lose the other, too.

The police's case crumbled in the face of Andrew's diagnosis and, of course, they did not pursue charges against his sibling. The coroner was keen to get on with the inquest. I phoned him to ask if he would support an application for charitable funding towards the specialist help the family would need. His response was predictable.

'That is absolutely nothing to do with me!'

Well, it was worth a try.

I was finally able to write Andrew's post-mortem report and in it I repeated my advice that the family should consult a specialist about the possibility that other members might share the same disorder. I told the coroner's officer I was willing to explain this to them and, soon afterwards, I was visited by Andrew's parents.

Grief walking into my office is a familiar sight, but still it never fails to affect me. The office is a place where paperclips and lists and calendars are devoted to the smooth running of our daily lives and yet here is an emotion so immense that it mocks the most carefully planned filing system. I braced myself to be kind but clinical. They had not come here for inadequate expressions of sympathy.

In fact, Andrew's mother was experiencing huge anger. His father sat in silence almost throughout. I wondered if he was always silent or if grief had rendered him mute. The mother, tall, strong, athletic and used to getting her own way, now eased her pain by blaming me. Not in a rational way, because no one was to blame for anything here.

She refused, point blank, to accept the possibility of inherited disease in her family. Not one of her antecedents, as far back as she could remember, had suffered from muscular dystrophy.

I agreed that the gene could mutate spontaneously but pointed out that, in many cases of Becker's muscular dystrophy, the mother is the carrier. Needless to say, that upset her even more. I persuaded her to talk about her history.

She was one of two sisters. Her sister's sons, both in their thirties, showed no indication that they suffered from any muscle disorder. She presented this as proof that my theory was nonsense, but it simply made me suspect that Mrs Styler was a great deal less lucky than her sister. I asked if her father was still alive. She told me that he had died in a road traffic accident when she was very young; she could hardly remember him.

I asked if she knew anything about the accident.

Mrs Styler paused.

'Well, I was told that he made a really terrible mistake. He seems to have put his foot on the accelerator when he should have put it on the brake. And before you ask, my father was teetotal.'

Fatal behaviour which could be mistaken for drunkenness. Here were distant echoes across generations. I very gently wondered out loud if there was any chance that her father might have been suffering from undiagnosed Becker's MD.

She was very angry at this suggestion. When she had calmed down, I asked if she knew of any other unnatural deaths, perhaps far back in her family.

This time she hesitated.

'I always thought . . . well, my mother used to say there was a curse, but I thought the men of the family were just a bit accident prone; it's a personality thing. I mean, there was a story about my father's grandfather. He was a real character, apparently. But he died young. He fell off his horse as he was about to win a race . . .'

I am not a genetic counsellor and could only listen quietly as she went through the painful process of reinterpreting family history and mythology. Sometimes we are remembered for the way we die and not the way we live and, tellingly, this seemed to be the pattern in her family.

The interview had been a success, I told myself, as she finally agreed that the family should be tested and counselled.

Then, just as they were leaving, she asked me another question.

'If you're right about this gene . . . is there a risk that Andrew's baby son could have it?' she asked.

Easy. 'No.'

'And what about Ian?'

Ah. Ian was Andrew's brother. This was the question I'd been dreading.

'Possibly.'

'How possibly?'

I reluctantly had to tell her that the chance was 50 per cent.

'So I've cursed my own sons,' she said, very quietly. 'When I gave birth to them, I gave death to them as well.'

I tried to say that, in a way, this is true of every one of us. But she was too upset to listen. She asked for the name of a genetic specialist and I recommended one.

I bumped into him not long afterwards and so had a chance to ask about the outcome for the family.

'Very sad,' he said. 'The surviving brother turns out to have Becker's MD. Bad luck that the mother gave it to both sons. There are two daughters as well, and one's a carrier. She already has a son. Family hasn't had the boy tested yet; they say they don't want to.'

Genes are merciless. Mutations, although they are mostly revealed very early in life, can lie in wait for the young to reach their prime before striking. Andrew's younger brother had been unkind, teasing him about his declining powers, publicly outstripping and humiliating him on the football field and at parkour. I wondered whether he had already noticed the first small intimations of his own declining powers. Perhaps his cruelty had not been the manifestation of youthful bravado or fraternal competition, but of fear.

If Andrew's MD had not been detected, how typical of deaths in this age group his would have looked, apparently involving both a momentary act of violence and reckless, drunken behaviour. The typical young male death I see is caused in these circumstances and it is caused by a single stab wound, a single gunshot wound or, often, the single punch.

The single punch is never intended to kill but it can do so with ease, generally in one of two ways. Let's say that a couple of young men are outside the pub and one is very angry. The pub is important because not only does alcohol intensify the aggressor's fury, but it relaxes the victim's neck, and the failure of the neck muscles to hold the head firmly can contribute to the outcome.

The angry man lashes out at his victim – often not straight in the face but to one side. Say the aggressor is right-handed and the punch lands on the left side of the jaw or even the upper neck. The victim's head is jerked sideways and at the same time rotates to the right before it is jarred backwards. I have seen it many times on slow-motion replays of CCTV footage. This sudden, abnormal movement of the skull – especially the rotation – can tear the small arteries to the brain which run up through special holes at the edges of the vertebrae. This structure is supposed to protect the arteries, but during a rotation it may actually hold, drag or pull them. Once damaged, of course the arteries bleed. Usually, the bleeding tracks upwards into that area beneath the middle membrane around the brain – the sub-arachnoid space.

Sub-arachnoid haemorrhage can kill so suddenly that witnesses in court often describe how a victim 'fell to the floor like a sack of potatoes'. But death is not necessarily immediate. There can be a lucid interval, when the victim walks and talks and seems normal – while pressure is actually increasing inside the head, caused by the build-up of blood leaking from the artery. First there is a headache. Then neck stiffness. Then, nausea. Finally, consciousness falters.

The second way a single punch can kill is by causing a fall backwards on to hard ground. Andrew Styler wasn't punched, but this is how he died. His head accelerated during the fall as gravity pulled him down. And then came to an abrupt stop when it hit the pavement: this sound is usually described by witnesses as a 'sickening thud'. The skull has stopped, but inside it the brain carries on moving. The deceleration injury is usually on the opposite side of the head from the place the bruise or fracture is found: it is contra-lateral, more commonly known as *contra coupe*. Beneath the thick, fixed membrane immediately beneath the skull – the dura – the tiny veins are sheared away by the moving brain, causing a subdural haemorrhage. And because veins bleed more slowly than arteries, there may be an even longer and more deceptive lucid period.

People often assume that a fractured skull is a cause of death, but this is seldom if ever the case. It is the brain moving within the skull that can cause fatal injury.

I daresay every Saturday night hundreds of people take punches. Hundreds fall over, drunk or stoned. Very few die as a result but, when a death occurs this way, families always ask: why has this happened to us? Andrew's mother asked me that over and over again. However much detailed medical knowledge goes into understanding each death, however lengthy a post-mortem report, however long pathologists and detectives and specialists spend analysing the deceased and the circumstances, there is usually one very major factor in such deaths which is impossible to quantify or review scientifically. It is luck.

9

I have come to regard the thirties as the age of excess. Just when we are leaving the idiocy of youth behind but still enjoy its bloom, when there are few natural causes of death to threaten us, it is so often extreme behaviour that kills this cohort.

In the thirties, families are often started, homes purchased, huge financial burdens shouldered, careers broken or built – perhaps creating a level of stress that drives some to the extremes which prevent the completion of this decade. Or perhaps, for others, the occasional bout of reckless behaviour in their twenties has now turned into a habit. And, in order to retain its attraction, maybe that habit has become more extreme.

Gareth Williams was almost thirty-two when he died in 2010. He was a very intelligent man and he worked for the intelligence services: consequently, many secrets, real or imagined, surrounded his death and these have allowed a plethora of conspiracy theories to take root around the case known as 'The Spy in the Bag'.

He came from the small, close-knit Welsh island of Anglesey, and his family seems to have been very close, too. From early on it was obvious that Gareth was a maths prodigy. He had taken his O-levels by the time he was ten and at seventeen had graduated from Bangor University with first-class honours. The following year he was awarded an MSc in Computer Science from Manchester University. He was soon employed at GCHQ, the listening and interpretation centre based in Cheltenham that provides the British government with security information.

Gareth was physically slight, but strong. He was a keen cyclist and enjoyed rock climbing and fell walking but, at the end of a day spent outdoors with other climbers or walkers, he did not go drinking with them. He was musical and interested in the arts. He had recently attended the Victoria and Albert Museum's Grace Kelly exhibition. He had very few friends. His sister told the inquest that he was selective about associates and he certainly was a loner and an exceptionally quiet and introverted man with little social life.

Of course, from his earliest years, Gareth's academic ability had been unusual and he had been taken out of his year group to study with children and then students much older than himself. That cannot have been easy and we can perhaps assume he had learned to keep his head down. Whatever his private thoughts and feelings, reports of his character indicate that he seldom chose to share them.

One night, about three years before his death, while he was working at Cheltenham, Gareth's landlady was awoken by his screams for help and she and her husband ran to his aid. They found that, using fabric rather than rope or handcuffs (fabric which nevertheless cut deeply into his skin), he had bound his wrists to the bedposts and was now powerless to free himself.

They released him and he explained to them that he had been carrying out an experiment to see if he could escape. Despite the nature of his work, they did not believe him: they took this to be a sexual episode. He promised never to try something so dangerous again.

He left Cheltenham in April 2009, moving to London for

157

a three-year secondment to MI6. He had high hopes for his new job but was soon unhappy. At his inquest, his sister – and he seems to have been closer to her than to anyone – said that he did not fit in with the 'flash' or 'fast car' culture of other MI6 operatives. There are hints of unpleasant office politics.

There has been no statement from the security services about Gareth Williams's exact work. Allegedly, he was a cryptologist, and it has been reported that he was one of a team that received a significant award for work in cryptology while he was at GCHQ. When he moved to MI6, did he become a 'spy'? According to many reports, he was an expert hacker, but his work was now perhaps not entirely confined to the computer screen: an MI6 witness, name withheld, told the coroner at Gareth's inquest that he had been 'operational', working alongside two undercover agents.

But after only about a year in London, Gareth had persuaded his employers to allow him to return to Cheltenham. In fact, as so often, his death occurred at one of life's junctions. He was preparing to leave London in a week or so: his flat, although extremely tidy, had an air of systematic packing about it. And only one week before, he had returned from a business trip to the western USA.

Gareth's colleagues had flown home when their work was completed, but he had extended the trip into a holiday. It has not been revealed where he went or what he did during this time, but it appears he ran up a very large credit-card bill. I do not believe anyone has seen this card statement except his employers and it is not clear to me how they obtained it. But MI6 took the bill and paid it off, explaining at the inquest that this was because Gareth had footed a colleague's hotel expenses. Anyone who knows how large organizations work and has tried to claim expenses for others may well be surprised by this explanation.

Gareth returned from the USA on 11 August. His movements between then and 15 August are little documented or not revealed. However, there is CCTV footage of him at the Bistroteque Club on 13 August. This was the cabaret room attached to a fashionable, warehouse-style east London restaurant. Jonny Woo, an artistic, bohemian mix of comedian, actor and drag queen, was a frequent performer in what had become known as the 'tranny tent'. Gareth did not stay late: he was home before midnight and CCTV footage seems to confirm that he was home alone.

On 15 August, he went shopping. He has been captured on CCTV wearing the same clothes he wore the day before, a red T-shirt and chinos. At 2330 on this day, one of his mobile phones was effectively wiped: it was returned to factory settings and it is not clear if this was carried out remotely by someone else, or by Gareth himself.

On Monday, 16 August, he was due to start his last, brief stint at MI6 before transferring back to Cheltenham, but he did not show up for work. It perhaps speaks volumes that no one investigated his absence. His flat was a security services 'safe house' in Pimlico, and another operative, who was scheduled to move in after his departure, came to view the premises, as arranged, at 1900 that evening. There was no answer. The following day, Tuesday, he tried calling Gareth. No reply. And apparently no follow-up.

Gareth's sister eventually phoned GCHQ almost a week later, on the following Monday morning, to say that she had not heard from him for some time and was worried. Late that afternoon, someone from GCHQ called the police. It certainly appears that no one at his office in MI6 was sufficiently interested in his absence to raise the alarm. This yawning gap between Gareth's absence from work and the eventual discovery of his body drew great criticism later from both the coroner and Gareth's family. The head of MI6 only then apologized for their failure to show concern.

About forty-five minutes after Gareth was finally reported missing, PC John Gallagher arrived at the flat. The first thing he noticed was that the lights were on. The second was that a woman's wig of long, flaming and unnaturally red hair was hanging on the back of a kitchen chair.

The flat was in good order and there was no evidence of any break-in. Upstairs, in the spare bedroom, neat piles of towels and hold-alls indicated that packing had been in progress. A few clothes were tidily laid out in the master bedroom. Less tidily, a bathrobe and bed sheet were strewn on the floor.

PC Gallagher opened the door to the en suite bathroom. It was windowless and the lights were off. There was a very strong and very unpleasant smell. The room was hot. Oddly for August, the central heating was turned to high. And in the bath was a large, red North Face hold-all. Its zip was padlocked shut.

He tried to lift the hold-all but could move it only about seven inches. He noticed that some dark and extremely malodorous liquid was seeping through it. At which point, PC Gallagher called for help.

The bag contained the naked and decomposing body of Gareth Williams. He was lying on his back in a foetal position, knees to his chest and arms folded across his chest. Beneath him, inside the bag, were keys, two of them on a ring. These were later shown to be the manufacturer-supplied keys to the padlock.

I was the third pathologist to examine Gareth. I did so one month after his death. I can confirm that there was no sign of neck injury and no object had penetrated his body. Indeed, there was no evidence of any potentially lethal trauma at all. There was a bruise on his left forearm. Both his elbows had quite prominent abrasions at the tips and there was, arguably, slight abrasion to his inner left eye. No natural disease appeared to have contributed to his death.

Toxicology ordered by Ben Swift, the first pathologist, found evidence of GHB in Gareth's liver. GHB is hydroxy-butyric acid, better known as a date-rape drug. This information, of course, fuelled a great deal of speculation, but things are not so simple. GHB is a naturally occurring chemical found in decomposing bodies and the toxicologist warned that, because the concentration was so low in both blood and urine, its presence was easily explainable by the post-mortem changes.

There was food in Gareth's stomach and Ben Swift had only this most unreliable means to help him estimate the time of death. What little evidence existed seemed to confirm what everyone suspected, that Gareth had died some time on the night of 15/16 August, after 0100, when his last internet browsing, of fashion and tech sites, was recorded.

Ben, faced with a considerable degree of decomposition and the absence of any apparent injury, was unable to determine the cause of Gareth's death. He recorded it as: Unascertained.

Meanwhile, a second forensic pathologist was called in. Ian Calder, an expert on deaths in confined spaces, confirmed all Ben Swift's findings and reached the same conclusion.

It is not clear why the then coroner, Dr Paul Knapman, took the unusual step of asking me to perform a third post-mortem. Perhaps because there was by now a wide-spread assumption in the press that Gareth Williams had been bizarrely murdered.

After a careful examination of Gareth's body, I agreed that the precise cause of death could only, from the simple pathological point of view, be classified as 'Unascertained' because the decomposition left so many questions unanswered. But there is much more to a death than the pathology alone and, considering the whole situation, I felt that the probable cause of death was asphyxiation – although I had to agree that we should keep in mind the possibility that he might have been poisoned. The presence of poison, more than asphyxiation, would have pointed to something which the press was already completely sure was the case: the involvement of a second person. But the extent of the decomposition severely limited the ability of the toxicologists to identify any poison. Despite extensive efforts, they could say only that none had been found but they could not completely exclude the possibility that some had been present. By the lower level of proof, that is, on the balance of probabilities, it was acceptable to say that no poisons were present. But could this be established by a higher level of truth: that is, beyond reasonable doubt? No.

And here is the fork in the road. Were others involved? Did they murder Gareth and put him in the hold-all? Did they force him into it? Or did they watch him get into it for reasons unknown and then leave the flat after some sort of accident? This last possibility was widely touted when it became public that Gareth had attended Jonny Woo's gig in east London: in the vivid imagination of the media, the leap was a short one from attending an arty drag act to inviting someone home for a sex game which then went wrong.

Despite some initial misleading information, it emerged

that there was no forensic evidence of the presence of others in the apartment or on the hold-all or on the bath: only Gareth's DNA was identifiable. I understand that there may have been a very limited number of DNA samples that were impossible to profile. At the time of writing, there is some discussion about applying updated profiling techniques. But, until proved otherwise, it seems just as – perhaps more – likely that they came from Gareth rather than someone else. There were no fingerprints or footprints, not even Gareth's, in the bath itself. Forensically, then, it was impossible to confirm that anyone else had been in the flat at the time of Gareth's death.

While three similar hold-alls in the spare room were packed with their keys still in the padlocks, the four to the hold-all Gareth died in had been separated. Two were found under his body, inside the bag. The other two were locked in a cashbox on his bedside table. There was no DNA or fingerprint evidence that anyone else had handled them. But no DNA means no genetic evidence. No ability to reach a conclusion. And, of course, the absence of evidence cannot be used to establish the evidence of absence.

Some believe that the high temperature in the flat shows that a visitor turned up the heating before leaving, deliberately hastening decomposition in an attempt to confuse pathologists. For the record, the daytime temperature on 15 August 2010 peaked in London at 22 degrees Celsius but had dropped to only 13 degrees by midnight. Gareth had recently returned from the sultry western United States, so it is not impossible that he was cold and fired up the heating himself.

Homicide theories abound, as always if there is a vacuum of real evidence. The most popular in this case is that, in the course of his work, Gareth had hacked into places where his presence was unwelcome and where he gained knowledge which threatened others. There is speculation that the British government, specifically, his own employer, may be included on the list of suspects. There are claims that he was protecting British banks from cyber-laundering and therefore terrorists or unknown foreign powers killed him. One theory is that his elimination served Israeli or Afghan interests. And Russian involvement was widely suspected when, five years after Gareth's death, a Russian agent who defected to the UK announced that his government had tried to recruit Gareth as a double agent. He said Gareth had refused the offer but, as a result of its being made, he was in possession of too much information about other double agents and therefore was eliminated by operatives who injected undetectable poison into his ear.

I am never sure why the relatively avascular ear – or the similarly bloodless space between the toes – is always the suggested route for these fatal injections. Maybe there is an assumption that pathologists do not bother to look in such boring, mundane areas of the body? Wrong. We do look everywhere, including the ears, the toes and anywhere else you care to mention.

All these theories were subsequently investigated, and that investigation itself seems to have been the subject of considerable turf wars between the security services and various parts of the Met.

But there was another area of the case to explore. Gareth's personal life.

I think the following details should be considered. Here is a different kind of post-mortem examination, a psychological one, but it may be just as revealing.

Gareth had attended two evening courses in fashion design at St Martin's and had in fact spent thousands on the designer dresses which hung in his wardrobe at the time of his death. He was a small and wiry man, 173 centimetres tall and weighing little over 60 kilograms. His BMI was only 20. I do not know the exact size of the dresses, so I cannot tell how well or if they would have fitted him, but, since all but a few remained pristine in their original wrapping, I think it is the possession but not the wearing of them which may be important.

He also had twenty-six pairs of expensive (many designer-made) women's shoes. Most were wrapped and pristine like the dresses: only four pairs had ever been worn. They were size 6½, apparently not too small for him, but they may have been tight. Again, what does possession rather than use tell us about the man and his life?

There were many feminine wigs in his flat, all locked into hold-alls similar to the one in which his body was found, apart from the wig the police officer found hanging on the back of a kitchen chair.

There were also make-up and accessories, none of which had been used.

There was DNA evidence of semen deposition – Gareth's semen only – at various places around the flat. None of it was on the dresses. Some was on the bathroom floor, beside the bath.

He had used and returned to four bondage/fantasy/fetishist websites in the previous year. At one bondage site, registration was required. Gareth evidently did have an interest in bondage, but there is no sign that it ever involved another party. One of his favoured sites was devoted to a niche pursuit: the fantasy of being restrained in a tight space and then escaping from it.

To many, this may seem a mysterious practice. Its root lies perhaps in a need to experience fear, even terror, to attain sexual satisfaction. Adrenaline is now widely associated with fight-or-flight responses but, before its sanitization by the Victorians, it had a broader nickname: it was called the 'fight, flight or frolic hormone'.

Both sides of the autonomic nervous system – those nerves we cannot control at will – are necessary to reach sexual orgasm. First the parasympathetic system, which is sometimes known as the 'rest and digest' system, relaxes and even comforts the body so that sexual stimulation is possible. Once excitement is established – and in the case of males this usually means an erection – the sympathetic system steps in. This results in the secretion of adrenaline, among other hormones, making the pulse race, causing tiny blood vessels to constrict, blood pressure to increase, and breathing to become heavy. For someone with severe coronary artery disease engaging in sexual activity, this can be a danger point. I have seen a number of deaths associated with this momentary massive boost of adrenaline, many of which, it must be said, occurred in an extra-marital situation. Death can, and surprisingly often does, result from an arrhythmia caused by that explosion of hormonal and neural activity which is orgasm. After orgasm, the parasympathetic system takes over from the sympathetic, resulting in a period of calm and often sleep.

The ways that people behave to increase adrenaline for extra sexual stimulation are many and varied. The use of methods of arousal outside what some people call 'normal' is known as paraphilia, and its sweep is broad. Some dressing-up might be at one end of the spectrum while, at the other end, could be restriction in a small place from which failure to escape is life-threatening. Autoerotic paraphilias are widespread and mostly entirely harmless. Until things go wrong.

Websites devoted to paraphilia, however risky their content, nearly always include serious health warnings, and I reiterate these. There is, by definition, seldom anyone around to help in the event of an emergency so there should be a fail-safe, a last resort, to ensure that it is possible to get out of trouble if necessary. Of course, knowing there is a safety net may lessen the excitement of the high-wire act and perhaps that is why, in the autoerotic deaths I have seen, some fail-safe systems were half-hearted or simply inadequate. Others were well designed and have clearly worked in the past but, for whatever reason, have not done so this time. I daresay there are plenty of effective fail-safe systems out there, but those are, of course, not the ones I see.

Asphyxiation may be the most perilous variation, usually involving plastic bags or hanging; this last accounts for 70 to 80 per cent of all autoerotic deaths. Many males have died this way, and a few women. So few that an apparent autoerotic death in a woman must be regarded with the utmost suspicion.

Perhaps it is chance alone which sometimes turns autoeroticism into a lethal practice. Maybe a change of material, of knot, or just the position of the ligature compressing the arteries of the neck alters everything. So that, instead of achieving, for that individual as so many times before, the slow drift into a state of pleasant, altered consciousness, there is rapid, catastrophic unconsciousness.

When oxygen supply is severely reduced to the brain, it is said to heighten all sensations, including, for some, erotic sensations. But, almost by definition, this pleasure is accompanied by a loss of control as consciousness fades. Some people even experience hallucinations. Not a good situation to be in when your life depends on your management of events. The intention is usually to slacken any constrictive device before consciousness slips too far. As consciousness fades, the grip on, for instance, the rope, should loosen and pressure on the neck should be relieved. That is the theory of many autoerotic practitioners, but my forensic experience proves it doesn't always work.

Psychologists tell us that there are three components of paraphilia: planning, the act itself and reliving it afterwards. And this third component of gratification used to be the hardest to achieve. Photographs and cine film were a preferred method, but few wanted to take their film to the local chemist's or photographic shop for development. However, the arrival of the mobile phone has changed everything. And the apparently widespread use of cameras in erotic and auto-erotic acts has given us new insights into this otherwise secret area of human behaviour. The interested professional can now see how long it takes for consciousness to fade. And, thanks to one near disaster during the filming of sado-masochistic pornography, which has now featured in textbooks in a way its makers could never have intended, we have learned a lot about the possibilities of reviving the asphyxiated.

Let's start the stopwatch when the camera films the star of the pornographic movie stepping off a chair with a classic noose around her neck. She hangs in complete suspension, feet off the ground. When fourteen seconds have passed, she appears to try to get back on the chair. Her right foot cannot reach it – and one second later her left foot fails, too. By fifteen seconds, she has lost consciousness. Her body arches backwards and her right foot kicks the chair away because by sixteen seconds she is having tonic-clonic convulsions – seizures, or fits, which make her whole body shake and move. By seventeen seconds, her arms stiffen and fold in at the elbows. The hands clench, the feet flex downwards. These are signs usually only seen in the neurosurgical intensive care unit, where they indicate significant anoxia in the more advanced, 'human', part of the brain, the cortex. The porn star must now be significantly deprived of oxygen, and those brain cells have stopped working properly. Technically, she is decorticate.

By eighteen seconds, her chest and abdomen are heaving, showing that her attempts at breathing are becoming desperate. And now, thankfully, a man in the room has realized this is not part of the show and that something is very wrong.

He grabs the rope and lets it down, but the woman's feet are not on the floor until the stopwatch shows forty seconds. By forty-four seconds, she is lying prone, the noose is loosened and there is no longer any constriction to her neck. However, by forty-five seconds, things are not getting better; in fact, they are getting worse. She is presenting a different pattern of positioning in her arms and legs. Her strange, contorted posture shows that lack of oxygen has spread from the sophisticated outer human cortex to the ancient brain within, the part that controls the heartbeat and breathing.

Her body is now rigid, legs and feet turned in, elbows extended. The hands are distinctive. They point in and back at the same time, like a maître d' accepting a tip. This is decerebrate rigidity. In an intensive care unit, someone would long ago have pressed the alarm button.

You might think that there can be no return from this.

Many doctors probably believe exactly that. But at fifty seconds, her decerebrate rigidity has taken a step backwards and has returned to decorticate rigidity and, by seventy-six seconds, her body has relaxed into a neutral position again. Incredibly, at ninety seconds, the star of the show regains consciousness. She gets up and walks away with, apparently, no ill effects. A very lucky lady. Alone, she would undoubtedly have died.

From this we understand that asphyxiation can be surprisingly reversible. Other studies of recorded autoerotic deaths show that the timing of the porn star's stages of asphyxiation are fairly typical, although for some people the whole process is much faster: the average loss of consciousness can start at ten seconds. Some are even unconscious in under five seconds. You can just never be sure.

Without a rescuer, without a fail-safe, when does death actually occur? Not long after loss of consciousness, that's certain. These recordings reveal that the body may continue to twitch randomly for an average of three to five minutes. Does the last twitch indicate the end of life? We don't know. What we learn is that hanging, or any kind of asphyxiation, may bring about a rapid loss of consciousness, which is not the same as a quick death.

It seems that the brief period of hypoxia just before loss of consciousness is both very exciting and extremely dangerous for those in search of autoerotic adventures. Most therefore plan self-asphyxiation in detail, and planning may bring its own gratification. In one case, a man had bolted his boots to a huge metal floor plate, tied a noose around his neck and attached the other end of the rope to his automated garage-door mechanism. That's a lot of planning. By holding the zapper, he could control the pressure on his neck. We will never know if he lost consciousness and had a seizure: we do know that, after several controlled movements of the door mechanism, for some reason the zapper fell out of his hand. On to the floor and beyond reach. He had no fail-safe, the garage-door motor could not be stopped. For several seconds, he continued to try to press the now imaginary button on the zapper that he still thought – hoped – was in his hand. Not a good end to a life. And total devastation for his family.

Forensic pathologists have seen fetishes of all kinds, but we see only those which have proved fatal. And we have learned that, when autoeroticism results in death, except perhaps in the case of teenagers, this is seldom a first attempt. The fatal act is generally at the end of a long line of safely completed but escalating adventures. Like any addiction, more and more is needed to achieve the same effect. And so satisfaction becomes dependent on the fantasy's increasing complexity. Until, in the end, complication occasionally proves fatal.

Forensic psychologist Anil Aggrawal has made a study of levels of fetishism. First, he says, comes desire, expressed perhaps as a light preference. Next, craving: a need to use that feature if at all possible. So a fetish is born. At the third stage, sex is not possible *without* the fetish. Finally, the object of the fetish takes the place of a sexual partner and, crucially, the slightest touch or scent may be sufficient to start, and perhaps complete, the process.

Paraphilia is widespread, maybe because the religious and moral issues which once burdened sexual activity are now a less heavy weight for most people. In a world where everyone is encouraged to explore their own sexuality, you might think there is no shame attached to bondage or other fantasies. But for many relatives of those who die this way, there is great shame.

On arriving at the scene where a lone man has died in circumstances that are less than clear, I have often found myself wondering if the family (having discovered Dad hanging when they return from a day out, or a teenager's body in his room in the morning) delay their shock for long enough to hide evidence like pornography or cross-dressing. Rather than admit to an autoerotic death, many would prefer a verdict of homicide, or even suicide, to public knowledge of the truth. And sometimes it really can be hard to differentiate an autoerotic accident from a suicide if the mechanics have left little possibility of survival and if there is no ancillary evidence of a sexual component. The absence of a suicide note, the presence of pornographic literature, evidence that the deceased has tried to pad the ligature to ensure it does not leave a tell-tale injury – these may all point to an autoerotic death but, even so, many remain as open verdicts, heard as the first or only case of the day in the coroner's court in order to avoid the press.

There seems to be a fairly widespread belief that, when the secret services carry out a homicide, they are in the habit of disguising their involvement as a lone, autoerotic accident or a suicide. Which brings us back to Gareth Williams. The murder investigation turned up no suspects and was beset with red herrings. Presented with the binary options of accident or murder, the police decided to establish whether it really was possible that he had climbed into the bag, zipped it and then padlocked it without help.

Their two confinement experts – a speciality you may not have known existed – attempted to climb into an identical bag, zip it up and then padlock it. These middle-aged men did not succeed – but both were larger, vertically and spherically, than Gareth, so I am disinclined to accept their evidence as proof. A young woman, shorter than Gareth but with his athletic physique, subsequently showed on YouTube that she could get into the same bag in under fifty seconds. It took her a further two minutes to zip it and lock it from the inside.

The investigation into Gareth's death was taking a long time and getting nowhere, and I doubt the internecine wars helped much. Dr Paul Knapman retired and Dr Fiona Wilcox replaced him as coroner. She felt she could delay an inquest no longer. There was no jury and much of the time there were no witnesses – the Foreign Secretary, William Hague, had signed a Public Interest immunity certificate releasing MI6 from answering certain questions on the grounds of national security. A few MI6 colleagues and staff did give evidence, and they sat behind a screen.

If you consider autoeroticism a source of great shame, and the indications are that Gareth's family did, then their suffering at the inquest must have been immense, as very private details about him were publicly aired. Of course, there was a lot of interest in the women's clothes found in his flat, even though a female friend who gave evidence said she believed that the dresses and shoes were intended as gifts for her or for his younger sister, Ceri.

Ceri concurred with that. She was also a witness and became something of a fashion icon during her appearances. She evidently adored her brother and her description of him included the information that he was profoundly risk averse. When mountaineering, he prepared carefully with maps and equipment checks. He would turn back, she said, even when very close to the summit, if he judged conditions unsafe to continue.

It was hard to reconcile this lovingly offered version of Gareth with the Gareth who might have taken such an immense risk by padlocking himself, naked, into a small bag. Evidently the coroner found such a reconciliation impossible. Dr Wilcox gave a narrative verdict which set out the details of the case. It made headlines.

She said that it was unlikely Gareth's death would ever be satisfactorily explained but, on the balance of probabilities, she concluded that he had been killed unlawfully and that his death was likely to have been 'criminally mediated'. She said that she thought he was alive when he got into the bag but was 'satisfied so that she was sure' that 'a third party' had moved the bag into the bath and that 'on the balance of probabilities' they had also locked the bag. She added that the question of secret service involvement in Gareth's death was a legitimate line of inquiry.

This verdict was a gift to conspiracy theorists. Gareth's suffering family immediately called for further investigation and the Met's homicide division continued to work on the case for another year. Finally, they announced that, although they could not 'fundamentally and beyond doubt' rule out the involvement of another party, they now believed that it was possible for Gareth to lock himself in the bag, that he had done so alone and died accidentally.

Other theories will never go away but, based on my own knowledge of this and similar deaths, I personally support the Met's final conclusion. Looking broadly at the man himself, there is no evidence that he intimately involved other people in his life. And there is no evidence that anyone else had even been in his flat. It is hard to believe that an attempt to clean up evidence of such contact would not have wiped away Gareth's prints and DNA as well.

Anyone who has ever tried to manipulate the dead, or even simply the unconscious, will know how immensely hard it is to move such a weight. Let alone fold that person neatly into a hold-all – there are reports that as many as nine people are needed to turn an unconscious Covid patient in ICU. I do not believe there is any likelihood that someone killed Gareth and then put him in the bag, certainly not without leaving a bruise on the body. As for carrying a 60-kilo man upstairs and into the bathroom in such a bag: well, most of us struggle with a 20-kilo suitcase when we go on holiday. Even two strong men would have had the greatest difficulty with such a dead weight in the hold-all, let alone lifting it into the bath. In my experience, lifting a toddler into a bath is hard enough.

There is no positive evidence of anyone else's involvement. But there is evidence of Gareth's interest in restraint. Although it is glossed over by many, I draw a direct line between his landlady finding him tied to the bed in 2007 and the police finding him curled inside a bag in 2010. In his flat, I sensed a neat and tidy – possibly overly tidy – man. But his semen deposits around the place spoke of someone for whom sex, entirely alone, was more exuberant. That it was an act through which he perhaps expressed his independence.

His sister said that he was a careful and risk-averse planner. She did not say he would never do anything risky, just that he carefully planned for that risk. He is likely, therefore, to have carried out a risk assessment and evidently he believed that, before either lack of oxygen or carbon dioxide build-up overwhelmed him, he would have time to unlock and unzip the bag. His grounds for such confidence may have been that he had managed successfully to do this in the past. We will never know.

At first appearances, locking and unlocking a soft bag from the inside may seem impossible. In fact, it is not difficult to create a hand-sized opening in a soft bag even where the two opposing zips are held together by a padlock. Airport thieves have been doing it for years. This has been demonstrated to me in training, when being warned about the risks to baggage at airports, and Gareth may very well have encountered it in training, too.

It is easy to close such a padlock, but a key is needed to open it. And the keys were found underneath Gareth's body. Why was that? Having escaped in the past, was he now so confident that he decided to set himself a more stimulating challenge by throwing in the keys before he climbed in himself? Or was this an error? A risk he had not considered or planned for? Did he simply drop the keys by mistake once he had padlocked the bag? I give some significance to the quite severe abrasions on both of his elbows, injuries that were typical of material burns, exactly the sort of injuries he would get by struggling desperately to recover the keys. As consciousness slipped away. And he considered the dangers of just one risk too many.

Many of the anomalies surrounding this case appear suspicious because the investigation has been dogged by secrecy. I know that conspiracy theories are more interesting for some. But, for me, Gareth Williams's very sad death fits into a pattern I recognize in the thirties age group. A pattern of managed but progressive risk-taking over the adult years has been escalated in order to achieve the same effect – until through bad luck or poor planning it now proves fatal.

Gareth's sexual interests harmed no one but himself, as far as we know. The manner of his death does not diminish in any way his achievements in life, which were considerable.

It does not impugn his brilliance or his character, widely described as generous and kind. The sexual side of his life was private and highly personalized, as it is for almost all of us: but in his case, I believe this, unfortunately, led to a tragic accident.

10

I walked into a flat in a very expensive London postcode and the first thing I noticed was not the body of the deceased but the smell of alcohol. The police thought they had a murder on their hands and forensic teams were busy, but one thing they could not swab was that tell-tale smell.

The flat was in a beautiful mansion block but, inside, it was squalid and dirty. It could not be described as chaotic because it was almost empty. There was just one chair, pushed against a wall, as if the occupant could seldom be bothered to sit down. The chair was surrounded by bottles, some standing, most on their side. It looked like the overflow that surrounds a full bottle bank on a Monday morning. Whisky, gin, a mysterious liqueur from Eastern Europe, wine, one bottle still a quarter full. And there were six tins of Special Brew, oddly crushed, as if someone had lain on them.

In a corner of the room was a large cabinet. Its doors were wide open and out of it spilled life's necessary but tedious paperwork – bills, statements, ominous letters in brown envelopes. Most were unopened and had apparently been chucked at the cabinet, many missing completely or bouncing straight out, so that the floor, in that corner only, was littered.

Near the centre of the room lay a woman of indeterminate age – I thought she might be fifty but was later informed that she was thirty-five. She was covered in bruises, especially around the genital and anal area. She wore high boots. Nearby lay bondage belts.

A detective saw me looking at all this.

'When we nick him, he's going to argue that it was consensual sex.'

'I doubt she consented to die,' I said, stooping to take her temperature.

'Wonder what she charged him?' a CSI nearby wondered out loud.

'Not a lot,' a young detective said. 'Have you seen what passes for a bed in the other room?'

Sex workers are, of course, extremely vulnerable, but the senior investigating officer shook his head.

'We don't know for certain that she was a prostitute.'

'Looks like it,' someone else said. 'Shitty rooms but a posh address to work from.'

I examined the woman. Her face was puffy and its colour was a red-purple that rarely occurs in nature, except perhaps in a stormy sky at sunset. Her cheeks were bloated. The left was distorted where it had been pressed hard against the floor. Her injuries were nasty but did not look life-threatening.

'No food in the kitchen,' another CSI told us. 'Nothing to eat at all.'

'Just bottles, then?' I asked.

She nodded. 'Empty ones.'

In the mortuary, the smell of alcohol when I opened the body was almost overwhelming. All the observers took a step back.

An officer now supplied the deceased's name: 'Felicity Beckendorf.'

I recognized that.

'Aren't Beckendorfs some sort of upmarket jewellers?'

'That's her family. Parents in Belgravia, brother in Manhattan.'

'Didn't see many jewels around her place,' observed another detective.

'She'd have pawned them for a bottle of whisky,' they all agreed.

I looked at Felicity's purple face. Her eyes were buried in the swelling, her features blurred by bloating. As soon as I had seen her in the apartment, I had felt that hers was a tragic case. Here was a woman who had allowed herself to be soundly beaten, either for money or in a search for sexual pleasure. Although, could she really have enjoyed receiving such brutal and violent treatment? And would her alcohol consumption have anaesthetized her to pleasure as well as to pain?

Take a sip of alcohol and it rushes down to the stomach and on to the small intestine: this is its principal site of absorption. It passes through the lining of the intestine straight into the bloodstream, where it travels rapidly around the body, most importantly to the brain. So absorption is the first step to drunkenness. However, at the same time, the alcohol reaches the liver and the process of elimination begins. Drunkenness, more scientifically described as the concentration of alcohol in the blood at any one time, is a constantly changing balance between absorption and elimination.

We absorb alcohol at different rates, and this is true of each individual at different times. For instance, alcohol disperses through the body's liquids but is almost insoluble in fat. Result: the overweight will probably have a higher blood alcohol level than lean drinkers after consuming the same amount. So will women, who naturally and healthily carry more fat than men.

Before it passes through the intestinal lining into our bloodstream and our brain, alcohol is often delayed in the stomach. If the stomach is entirely empty, it would take the small intestine about ten minutes to absorb 100 per cent of it. But if taken with, or after, food, its progress is delayed until this has been sufficiently digested. If that food is fatty or milky, the delay may be longer.

The strength of the alcohol is obviously an important factor in absorption: sherry, port, gin and tonic or, my own favourite, whisky and soda, have an alcohol content of about 20 per cent and so have high rates of absorption. Beer is absorbed much more slowly: its sheer volume gives the alcohol in it less access to the gastric lining and therefore the bloodstream. And it is full of carbohydrates, which further delay absorption: if you dilute whisky to the same strength as beer, it will still make you feel more drunk more rapidly.

The body itself tries to delay its absorption of very strong drink. The muscle movements pushing the alcohol through the digestive system may slow and the gastric lining can become so irritated that it produces a thicker mucus barrier, which causes delay. With so many different factors affecting the absorption rate, it is very hard to give a rule of thumb, but a rough guideline is that 60 per cent of alcohol consumed is absorbed within sixty minutes.

So what about the other part of the drunkenness equation, the body's elimination of alcohol? This is almost entirely down to the liver and is a much less variable process. But some people have larger livers, women eliminate alcohol slightly faster than men and, as usual, genes have a role to play. Certain genes cause a drinker to experience unpleasant side-effects like flushing and nausea long before happiness, bonhomie or euphoria kick in. For anyone with these genes – and they are most likely to be found in Jewish and East Asian populations – drinking alcohol triggers immediate suffering.

Consequently, such genes are regarded as protective against alcohol dependency, although environmental factors are still highly significant. When social drinking increased substantially in 1980s Japan, a study found that the percentage of alcoholics carrying a protective gene also increased, and by more than four times.

The liver's enzymes eliminate alcohol by putting it through a three-part oxidization process until it becomes little more than carbon dioxide and water. How long does this take? The findings are many and various. A very regular drinker, indeed, the chronic alcoholic, can eliminate as much as three times faster than the occasional drinker. 'Units' of alcohol are a health education invention, not a scientific measure (they are equivalent to about 8 g of pure alcohol in the UK: in the USA, one unit is about 14 g). Very roughly, one unit can be eliminated by one adult in one hour. A unit in the UK is half a pint of beer, a single shot of spirits or a small glass of wine. Government advice for both men and women is to drink less than fourteen units a week and to give the busy liver recovery time by keeping some days drink-free.

Units do seem to have an almost magical elasticity. I am referring to the ability of the human mind to underestimate dramatically the number of units consumed the previous week or yesterday or even tonight. While we are drinking, the organ which should be making a rational decision about our blood alcohol level is, unfortunately, greatly affected by it. Alcohol is swiftly carried to the brain by the blood and readily passes through the blood/brain barrier. Very soon, nerve cells are bathing in white wine and behaving rather strangely, a sensation many people enjoy.

Alcohol's effects on neurons is similar to a lack of oxygen: it turns them off, or at least slows them down. Blood alcohol levels are measured in milligrams of alcohol per 100 milli-litres of blood. At 30 mg/100 ml some people begin to find that this slowing of the neural network means they become disinhibited. Complex skills (including driving) may show some initial impairment. At 50 mg/100 ml, many more people experience this. The limit for blood alcohol concen-tration when driving in Scotland is 50 mg/100 ml: in the rest of the UK it is 80 mg/100 ml. However, by this stage, some drinkers (especially if they are unused to alcohol, have not eaten or have a high percentage of body fat) will already be feeling distinctly squiffy. Most will have experienced loss of inhibition to some degree and found themselves talking – and, we hope, laughing – more than usual.

At this level of concentration, it is the more sophisticated, specialized cells of the cerebral cortex that are affected. But if drinking continues at a rate where absorption greatly exceeds the liver's ability to eliminate, the concentration rises and the depressant effect reaches the nerve cells of the mid-brain. So at 100–150 mg/100 ml, words may be slurred, walking becomes harder and some may begin to feel sick.

By 200 mg/100 ml, many are vomiting. Walking has prob-ably become an uneven stagger. Speech may not be entirely comprehensible to others.

At still higher concentrations, stupor and sometimes coma results, because nerve cell inactivity is spreading to the medulla – the ancient part of our brain which, independent of any instructions from the boss, controls our vital actions. Anyone, even a habitual drinker, who reaches 300 mg/100 ml is in danger of dying. The drunk often suffer fatal trauma: many a homicide is triggered by alcohol aggression and road traffic accidents are much more common. Other calamities might include falling downstairs, burning in a fire started inadvertently, hypothermia caused by falling asleep in the park on a freezing night, drowning, perhaps by tumbling into the river when stopping to urinate on the way home and, of course, inhaling the inevitable vomit as unconsciousness and gastric irritation collide.

When, as a keen young pathologist, I travelled the length and breadth of London carrying out many post-mortems per day on sudden but non-suspicious deaths, I arrived at each mortuary to find not only the usual strokes and heart failures but a roll-call of deaths by drunkenness. The World Health Organization calculates that over 5 per cent of all deaths worldwide are associated with alcohol and that in the twenty to thirty-nine age group an amazing 13.5 per cent are 'attributable to alcohol'. And it may not be the fight, the stairs, the fire, the cold, the river or the vomit that kills the vulnerable drunk: it may well be the alcohol itself.

Above a concentration of 300 mg/100 ml, the nerve cells deep in the brain that control our heart and breathing are in something close to torpor. The heart rate may now be so slow that oxygen-carrying blood is not reaching vital organs. Or the brain may be incapable of recognizing that carbon dioxide is building up and so deeper breathing is necessary to take in more oxygen. So as consumption continues to rise past this level, death is at first a serious possibility, then a probability and then inevitable.

I would have no idea, until the tox report came back, just how much Felicity Beckendorf had drunk. That she was a regular consumer of huge quantities was not in doubt. Her liver did not have the healthy appearance of a sleek stingray gliding through the ocean; it was more like something shrunken and corroded, covered in pits and barnacles, which has lain a long time on the seabed. Alcohol, wisely used, can be life enhancing for some, but regular drinkers must steer a course between the capacity of this drug both to improve life and to shorten it. As well as causing liver damage and cirrhosis, it is a significant risk factor for many different types of cancer. It is also strongly associated with high blood pressure, which can result in heart disease, probably dementia and definitely strokes.

My friend Simon, whose parents had heaved a sigh of relief when he passed his A-levels and reached medical school, did qualify to become an anaesthetist. We remained on good terms once we started in our different specializations but, as time went on, we saw a lot less of each other. I told myself this was because we were both very busy. Maybe I should have admitted that the real reason was that I could not keep up with his drinking. I was very far from teetotal, but seeing Simon meant drinking such vast amounts, or watching him do so, that it had started to be a rather uncomfortable experience.

One day Simon was on call at the hospital and, when buzzed to an emergency, he did not respond. I am sorry to say that he was found in a drunken stupor and sacked on the spot. His misery did not last long. Very shortly afterwards, he had a stroke and died instantly. He was thirty-two.

Youthful strokes occur more often than you might think, but they may have a different cause from those which occur in old age. Most are associated with bleeding from an arterio-venous malformation. An AVM is a congenital abnormality that bears a striking resemblance to a bird's nest or the knotted, tangled lengths of string you find at the back of a kitchen drawer. It consists of a ball of blood vessels: tiny arteries, veins and even sometimes a strange anatomical hybrid of the two, all twisted together in a sort of mass. They may form in other places in the body, like the nose or liver or spleen, but they most often cause serious problems in the brain. Occasionally I have found them in the brains of old people who have died of something unrelated: they have nestled there for more than eighty years and caused no problems. These people are winners in life's fickle lottery because usually the presence of such an odd tangle of vessels is a great weakness in the brain's circulation. And at some point – starting from, and perhaps particularly during, the thirties – they are likely to rupture and bleed.

At his post-mortem, Simon's stroke was indeed found to have been caused by a ruptured arterio-venous malformation. I still miss him, even now. There are times I laugh at something and I know Simon, of all people, would have laughed with me. Looking back, I can see that his depression and drinking must have had roots somewhere deeper than the days when a blonde tossed her hair around a lot. Maybe the home I regarded as such a happy one had not been so. But it is too late for such reflections. Part of ageing involves reconstructing the past, and that often means asking ourselves the questions we should probably have asked long ago.

Did Simon's drinking help cause the blood vessel rupture? Maybe. Excessive alcohol consumption is one factor that can put increased pressure on the genetic weakness of an AVM. So can cocaine use, which may cause a dramatic rise in blood pressure, but I don't think Simon ever graduated from his first love to another drug.

Despite the likely role of alcohol in his death, it would have been recorded in national statistics as a natural one. Only about 6,000 people in their thirties die each year in England and Wales, less than half the number who die in their forties, and the leading causes are not natural. Although an unnatural death, I was sure that Felicity Beckendorf's was not a homicide, and the police did stop their investigation, because her injuries were certainly not very serious. There was a chance of a stroke, like Simon, and I would investigate this, of course. However, I suspected that she conformed to statistics: the majority of deaths at this age are caused by accidents, suicide or alcohol misuse.

But the nature of that misuse is changing.

The twenty-first century has seen a decline, among the young, of deaths from alcoholic liver disease. This indicates that chronic drinking may not have become so established in the young of recent generations as in my own generation. But death by alcohol poisoning – essentially, binge drinking – tells a different story. And, as usual, death statistics reflect society's changes.

At the beginning of this century, pub closing time was rigorously policed and supermarkets had not started treating alcohol as a loss leader. When that changed, so did drinking patterns. Relaxation of the licensing laws meant that drinking was no longer an expensive and tightly regulated social activity. Shop-bought alcohol became so cheap that it has been, increasingly, consumed at home. And even those who usually drank outside the home before the recent pandemic lockdowns may well have established the home-drinking habit now.

I like to sit down in the evening with a whisky because I am, personally, a home drinker. That is something I share with the young but, for them, it's binge drinking at home. Alcohol-related deaths in the under-forties started to climb dramatically from 2011 as a result. All eyes are on Scotland, followed now by Wales, to see if their interesting experiment in social engineering can calm this increase. In 2018,

Scotland became the first country in the world to introduce a minimum price for a unit of alcohol: it was set at fifty pence per unit and it was estimated that, as a result, alcohol-related hospital admissions would fall by at least 1,500 per year.

So had Felicity Beckendorf died after one massive binge? Or because of long-term alcohol abuse, that is, drinking too much, too often? Her liver was certainly in a chronic state but perhaps not quite diseased enough to have killed her yet. I concluded it was most likely that she had died of acute alcohol poisoning from a night of excessive drinking. But was there some other reason?

Alcohol is a risk factor for a wide range of diseases and conditions. Among these is the most common cancer in the UK: breast cancer. In fact, of the risk factors for breast cancer that a woman can control, alcohol is the greatest. So, despite her youth, I was not entirely surprised to find, during my routine examination of her breasts, that the left contained something hard and white.

Breasts are principally yellow fat but through this runs the thin, white stringy tissue that contains milk-producing glands. The tumour was about the size of a marble and in my fingers it felt almost as hard. Its very whiteness, so different from the surrounding tissue, seemed threatening. With the naked eye alone, it was obvious that this should not be here.

Cancer is Latin for a crab, and this spreading, malignant tumour did look like a crab in her breast. Extending from the crab's round body and just as hard, interwoven with the fatty tissue and following the gland lines, were its legs and pincers: the threads of growing cells, dividing, reproducing, extending further and further. The pincers had already spread two centimetres and it is almost certain that Felicity would have noticed the lump. Had she chosen to prolong her life by visiting the doctor? I doubted it. Apparently, it had not yet metastasized to other parts of the body – liver and bone are the most likely site for secondary tumours – but it was probable that, without treatment, it would have killed her within a year.

Many cells in the human body are not remanufactured. You're born with them and, after reaching a certain age, usually the mid-twenties, these irreplaceable cells start to die. Our lifetime of lost cells, of biological ageing, this process of decline, this senescence, though we might fight it, is inevitable. But some cells *are* replaced, constantly.

Anywhere cells are actively reproducing is a possible primary cancer site. Skin cells are always in a state of replication, starting a few layers down and then moving towards the surface as old cells are sloughed off. Liver cells work hard to reproduce in order to fill any gaps left by last night's party (although Felicity's liver cells had long ago lost their battle against partying). And the cells of breast tissue reproduce, too. Replication of these cells is normal and, if controlled, entirely healthy. Excessive local replication may, sooner or later, lead to cancer.

I looked at Felicity's tumour on a microscope slide. Instead of neat patterns and rows of cells, reminiscent for me of a classroom at Watford Grammar, it seemed a maniac had flung all the desks around in chaotic heaps. We don't always know exactly what causes cells to start proliferating out of control, but we know that in breast tissue the cellular response to hormones is a very common trigger. The breast is targeted by countless different hormones through a woman's lifetime: when she reaches puberty; each month as her cycle of egg release begins again and again; then later, when she is pregnant; when she is breastfeeding; when she is menopausal . . .

the tide of hormones rises and falls, grows and recedes, its composition always subtly changing. Oestrogen and progesterone, made in the ovaries and, during pregnancy, in the placenta, are the best known, but there are others, including growth hormones, human chorionic gonadotrophin and prolactin. The ones which stimulate needed cell proliferation on occasions probably also stimulate unneeded and unwanted replication. They are the friend and the enemy.

Some scientists think that there could be times in a woman's early life – perhaps when she is a girl and breast cells are proliferating rapidly – when she could be especially susceptible to carcinogens which will later result in malignant changes. But there are many risk factors, and the majority are outside any individual's control. The biggest is being female – around 55,000 women in the UK are diagnosed with breast cancer each year, and just about 300 men. Age is the next most significant. A woman of fifty is ten times more likely to have breast cancer than a woman of thirty. Location apparently plays a role, perhaps through population genetics: breast cancer rates in north-west Europe are the highest in the world, with the Netherlands topping the list and the UK not far behind. The lowest rates are in East Asia and South America. This is a lifetime risk, so it may be that where you were born is as important as where you live now.

The chances of having breast cancer are higher if you belong to a population with a significant incidence of certain gene mutations. For instance, Ashkenazi Jews are more likely to carry two of the mutations linked to breast cancer, BRCA1 and BRCA2. Conversely, there are some populations that are much less likely to develop breast cancer. In the UK, black and Asian women may be as much as half as likely; studies vary. Other factors – many of which carry very low risks – include living in a city, being tall (over 165 cm), being wealthy (or advantaged), having a higher birthweight, starting menstruation early or menopause late and having no children or having them late in life.

One in eight women in developed countries faces the unwelcome diagnosis of breast cancer at some time. The good news is that survival rates have been improving substantially. But why are breast cells turning malignant in so many women around the world and why is the incidence of tumours increasing?

DNA is an amazing molecule. In fact, it is far too big for our needs as humans, so only parts of it are turned on at any one time. Through our lives, chunks of the DNA molecule are quite naturally switched on and off to allow for changes such as puberty or the menopause. But many bits of it are just gobbledygook and are never normally turned on at all.

This molecule is so crucial to our wellbeing that it is policed by special repairing enzymes in our cells. They aim to keep the DNA neat and pristine and functioning well. However, these policing enzymes are themselves derived from the DNA they are correcting. If there is an error in the piece that codes for them, they may fail to function properly. The self-repairing mechanisms can do a huge amount – but may not necessarily repair themselves.

DNA mutations might be inherited. Or the DNA may have been damaged by some environmental threat, like radiation. Or the changes may, of course, simply be spontaneous. The longer you live, the more opportunity there is for mutations to occur, which is why, broadly speaking, the risk of breast cancer increases with age. Felicity, at thirty-five, was part of a cohort that tells a different story. Breast cancer rates are rising. But it seems they may be rising faster in the young.

The number of newly diagnosed cases in younger women – and by that I mean under thirty-five – has risen at more than twice the rate of increase in older women over the last ten years. This is evident from the statistics available at the time of writing, which, unfortunately, are for England only. Maybe it is a blip, because statistics become less reliable with small numbers of cases, and these numbers are, thankfully, small. When explaining them, better screening must be taken into account. Regular mammograms are offered to all women in the UK between the ages of fifty and seventy, but those known to be at genetic risk are usually screened from thirty, and sometimes earlier. The breast tissue of younger women may be so dense that it cannot accurately be read by mammograms and so an MRI scan might be offered. This is a wonderful service, but I'm not sure it can fully explain the apparent rise in early breast cancer. Is it possible that lifestyle choices are increasing the number of cases among young women?

According to Cancer Research UK, about a quarter of breast cancer cases may be preventable. How, then, can a woman diminish her own risk? There are many suggested factors, most of which change the equation only slightly. Just as a high number of unfavourable lifestyle choices does not automatically lead to breast cancer, actively ensuring risks are reduced will not offer certain protection against a rampant gene mutation, whether spontaneous or inherited.

The greatest of these factors is alcohol, as Felicity demonstrates. All studies agree on this and, in fact, there seems to be no entirely safe level for alcohol consumption. It is currently unclear whether binge drinking does more harm than regular, lower-level drinking, as there has been little research in this area. Should a woman really stop drinking to lower her risk? Perhaps that depends on the impact this would have on her life and the full spectrum of risks she carries.

Weight is also a significant factor. Many people will be surprised to know that premenopausal breast cancer occurs less often in overweight women. A high BMI can create so many other health problems that the link between body fat and a decreased risk of breast cancer, particularly in the young, goes largely unpublicized. That link is probably explained by the body's suppression of some hormone production – which is one effect of storing excess fat. In fact, the overweight eighteen-to thirty-year-old lessens her risk of breast cancer for many years. However, for anyone who stays overweight right through adulthood, or who gains weight after the age of thirty, the birds do finally come home to roost after menopause. A high BMI throughout adulthood, and certainly a high BMI post-menopause, does increase the risk of breast cancer in later life.

We all know what a healthy diet looks like – low fat and lots of fruit and vegetables. In fact, although cutting down on fat or sugar has many other benefits, there is no evidence that it lowers the risk of breast cancer. However, the calcium in dairy products (supplements do not have the same effect) does help, and so does the consumption of fruit and vegetables over a lifetime and certainly for at least twelve years, particularly if their colour is green or orange.

As well as a good diet, we now think that exercise, sleep, a balance between stress and relaxation, social interaction and personal hygiene are all important to a healthy lifestyle. But this is a modern concept applied to controlling a DNA molecule which has been selected over millennia. Given the complexity of our current lives and diets, a molecule that initially supported a hunter's ability to run may not have such a beneficial effect nowadays.

I have listed some of the main risk factors for breast cancer, but my suspicion is that the disproportionate increase in this cancer in the young may be largely linked to one factor. This factor is reflected in a parallel rise in the death statistics of the young. I am referring to binge alcohol consumption.

When the tox report came back on Felicity's blood samples, it showed something astonishing. Her alcohol level at death was 540 milligrams of alcohol per 100 millilitres of blood. Given that the driving limit in England is 80 mg/100 ml blood and that one might reasonably be expected to die at 300 mg/100 ml blood, it is amazing that Felicity Beckendorf had survived cardiorespiratory failure long enough to keep consuming alcohol until she reached 540 mg/100 ml.

For cause of death, I gave acute alcohol poisoning. At that level, how could I give anything else?

I found her death a particularly sad one. A police officer told me they had learned she had, in fact, funded her drinking through prostitution when her family cut off all contact, emotional and financial. She appeared to have been born with every advantage, but her need for alcohol had robbed her of any self-respect and her death had been a painful and demeaning one. Or was it the other way around? Had traumatic events in her past created a chasm that she had found only drink could fill?

I wondered what the family fault lines could be that had shifted the tectonic plates in Felicity's life and led to her early death. Perhaps the family would indicate this at the inquest. But it was a sad, small affair. I gave evidence to the coroner and so did a junior police officer. No one else came. The Beckendorfs sent a statement to the court saying that they felt they had lost their daughter to alcoholism a long time ago: they had sent her to rehab several times but she had been unable to stop drinking and consequently there had then been no contact for some years. They were sorry to hear of her death but felt they could not help the court in any way.

I wrote to the police officer dealing with the case, asking him to inform the Beckendorfs of Felicity's breast cancer. Given its possible genetic component, it was right that they should know. Her cancer had not contributed in any way to her death, but it was an important finding because it might have been familial and therefore I included it in a post-mortem report that I daresay only the coroner bothered to read.

Felicity's drinking had become extreme at an early age. Probably she was very young when she became addicted and, for the young, adapting lifestyle to recognize risk is hard, because death's threat does not feel near. Many of us old enough to know better who are much closer to the consequences of long-term drinking still consume too much, so it is hard to imagine that the under-forties will easily review risks and change habits. For those in their thirties, extremes – of sexual or social behaviour – seem to carry few immediate consequences. They look around and see so many getting away with it. But, as we reach our forties, all that begins to change.

And then the justice;
In fair round belly with good capon lin'd,
With eyes severe and beard of formal cut,
Full of wise saws and modern instances;
And so he plays his part:

11

'When I met Zoe, it was love at first sight. We have been married for twelve years. Our marriage was good, in my opinion, until about a year ago, when she told me she had gone off sex.

'I did not believe Zoe was having an affair until the beginning of this month. She has beautiful red hair and everyone turns to look at her wherever she is. It was going a little bit grey at the temples and it didn't matter, and I didn't think she cared, but suddenly she started to dye the hair around her temples. I thought that was very odd. Then, once, when I came home from work and caught sight of her slipping into the bathroom, I thought I saw her wiping make-up off her face with a towel. I asked her and she denied it but, when I inspected the towel, I found clear signs of make-up on it. I suggested that she was seeing someone. She denied it. Then she said: "I don't love you any more, Mark." My younger daughter overheard and started to cry and no more was said.

'After work the next day, I asked her if we were going to stay together. She said that she loved me, but not in the way I wanted her to love me. We left it at that. The next morning we were both happy: she asked if I would like to meet her best friend. I said I'd like to meet her. And she said: no, it's a "him". Then everything fitted.

'I think maybe she had been having a relationship for a year. She said her friend was called Gary and that he was her best friend, he helped her and she can talk to him when she can't talk to me because I fly off the handle. She denied having a relationship. I know she was. I tried to go to work but was so upset that I had to come home.

'While Zoe was at work, I looked through her belongings and found Gary's phone number. I phoned him and he answered, and I said that I understood Zoe and he were the best of friends and wanted us to meet for a drink. I said that I was sorry but I did not think I could do that. He said that was okay, he was just there for Zoe when she needed him.

'I phoned Zoe at work at 1400, but she had already left. She did not get home until 1745. I believe she spent that time with Gary. And, I am not proud of my behaviour, but for about a month I had been checking her underwear in the evening and on about six occasions I had found semen in her knickers.

'The next day was Saturday. In the morning, when she thought I was having a bath, I saw Zoe sending a text. I asked if it was to Gary, and I looked at the phone and it said: "Don't worry, it will be okay." She said that Gary was just asking if she was okay. I told her about the evidence I had found in her underwear.

'On Saturday afternoon Zoe went to sleep and I went to see her parents and told them about her affair. Her father was livid. Her mum had to calm him down. Later, she saw Zoe, and Zoe cried and said she has a platonic relationship with Gary.

'The following week I noticed that there were other signs Zoe was having an affair, like doing her shopping online to give her more time. I really need the police to search Gary's house: they will find that she had been there and I am not going mad and I am not crazy.

'On Tuesday I went to work but left to follow Zoe because

she said she was going shopping. She had a meeting with Ruby's teacher, and then she would normally go to Sainsbury's. She did not go to Sainsbury's. She went to her sister's house. When she found she was out, she pulled away and headed down the main road. This leads to Waitrose, and it also leads to the town where Gary lives. I lost her in the traffic and, despite searching, could not find her car in the car park. Later, at home, she said that Waitrose was so busy she went back to Sainsbury's, and there were indeed Sainsbury's bags of shopping everywhere. I think she had seen me following her. But when I told her that is what I had done she told me to go and see a doctor and offered to make me an appointment. He prescribed some pills.

'That night I looked at our wedding photos and started to cry. Zoe woke up and I told her I could not be without her and the children. She said I wouldn't have to be without them. But I said that would happen because she didn't love me any more. She said she was very tired and wanted to go back to sleep. I went into the kitchen and I could not stop crying. I went over things again and again in my head and could find no solution. At 6 a.m. I woke Zoe and told her I had to talk to her. She said she was tired. I said I would make a cup of tea and went into the kitchen.

'I put the kettle on and, for some reason, I put the kitchen knife up the sleeve of my dressing gown and then went back into the bedroom. I woke Zoe again and told her that I could not live without her and that I would kill myself. I then took the knife out and put it to my stomach and looked into her eyes. She sort of half smiled. She almost smirked at me. She said: "You can't blame me!" She sat up and I pushed the knife into her stomach. She lay down and started breathing heavily. I got up and walked around. Then I picked up the phone by the bed and phoned my mother and told her I had stabbed Zoe.

'I can't remember what she said. I put the phone down and got on to the bed, and Zoe was asleep. I gave her a kiss and told her we would be together now. I put the blade to my stomach and tried to push it in. But I could not. I had to move it higher. Then I pushed it in and felt it go in. The phone rang just then and I still had the blade in me. I picked it up, and it was my mother and I told her to hurry. I dropped the phone and lay down on the bed next to Zoe.

'When the girls came in, I told them to go and watch the TV and that Mummy had gone out. The next thing I remember was my mother standing over me, and then I don't remember anything until the next day, when I awoke in hospital.

'I have been told that Zoe had several knife wounds, but I definitely remember stabbing her only once and then her going to sleep. I don't remember having any struggle with her. I remember the look in her eyes and on her face when she said: "You can't blame me." And I realized at that point that she did not care if I stabbed myself or not. I really do not think that she cared.'

As Zoe's body was wheeled into the post-mortem room, the mortuary assistant looked at me.

'No one can understand,' he said, 'how that geezer keeps insisting he only stabbed her once.'

I lifted the sheet. Zoe was an attractive woman in her forties with long, flaming-red hair, greying slightly at the temples. Her hair was the first thing you noticed about her, and that must have been true in life as well as death. I noticed it even before her many knife wounds.

'He's mad, that's how,' said the one police officer who was present. 'We think he'll get away with a manslaughter charge.'

Many police officers regard manslaughter as a very poor relation to murder. Still more see it as a loophole through which perpetrators, feigning insanity, can too often slip.

The mortuary assistant said: 'I suppose the husband only has to find a nice tame shrink to say he's bonkers and –'

'– and it's manslaughter. He'll be out in a few years,' the police officer agreed. 'I mean, why did he kill her? What's wrong with divorce? Here's two people with enough money, good jobs. Two kids . . .'

'What on earth's going to happen to those girls now that their mum's dead and their dad's going to jail?' asked the mortuary assistant sadly. We shook our heads.

Zoe had died two weeks ago. This was her second post-mortem. The first pathologist to examine a body has usually been called by the police and so will almost always be giving evidence for the prosecution. When charges are brought, the defendant's solicitors will generally ask for a second post-mortem. How different this is from the first. The room is much quieter and emptier because only one token police officer is likely to attend and perhaps no one else is there at all, just me and the mortuary assistants. The body has been dead for some time and, even with help from mortuary fridges or freezers, may be decomposing. Cuts and dissections have already been made, of course, and sometimes crucial organs will have been kept back for specialists to examine so something as vital as the brain or the heart may not be present.

The second pathologist is heavily reliant on photos, both from the original post-mortem and the crime scene. I had already examined pictures of Mark and Zoe's bedroom. They were a well-off professional couple. The room was large, airy and well ordered. There was a pair of fluffy slippers placed neatly at the bedside and make-up was arranged on small trays on the dressing table. But the bed was chaotic. The duvet was half on the floor and the rest of the covers were twisted as if a whirlwind had hit. None of them was red, but there was so much blood on them that they might have been. A different, brighter, more shocking red than her hair.

Zoe, wearing pale pyjamas, lay awkwardly. One arm was stretched out; the other half covered her body. Her head was back. Her position told me that she had fought for her life.

My first job was to examine her and so confirm the findings of my colleague. There can be disagreement between the two pathologists on the medical facts of a death, but this is unusual. Assuming the pathology can be agreed, it is the job of the defence pathologist to examine the facts afresh with a view to alternative interpretation.

I was able to identify all the wounds the report described. One injury to the neck, three to the front of Zoe's chest, four to the back of her chest, two in the legs and seven in the arms. In addition, post-mortem changes meant that, since my colleague had finished her work, further bruises had appeared on Zoe's legs, arms and back. None of it was helpful to the defence.

I admired my colleague's skilful dissection and the mortuary assistant's neat stitching, designed to be out of sight for relatives visiting the body. I had no choice but to cut through them to open Zoe's abdomen and, after the disturbance of the previous post-mortem, it was very hard to follow the tracks of the wounds. I did, however, notice how the spine had been nicked and the ribs had been severed in places, indicating the great force with which the knife had penetrated the body. Skin and muscle are quite easy to penetrate, but cutting through bone really does require some effort. No one can claim that the knife inexplicably slipped into the body if bone has been cut.

I agreed with the post-mortem report that death had most likely been caused by the injuries which penetrated the heart, aorta, liver and spleen. And I added that a couple more to the lungs were also potentially fatal.

The wounds on both arms were probably defensive injuries, and I calculated that an unusual cut on the right shin was also a defensive injury, inflicted during the struggle on the bed. There was evidence in every one of these of considerable movement between perpetrator and victim. Clearly Zoe had put up a fight and had not obligingly 'gone to sleep' after being stabbed just once, as her husband had described.

'Doubt you can help the defence much,' the police officer said.

He was right. I examined a picture of a bloodstained chef's knife which my colleague had measured at 20 cm long and 3.5 cm wide. It was the right size and shape to have caused the wounds.

In my report, I could do nothing but agree with the first pathologist that the injuries were entirely consistent with a sustained assault rather than with Mark's version of events. When two pathologists concur, there is no point calling both to the witness stand and I did not therefore go to Mark's trial. However, the solicitors kept me informed. The prosecution described Mark's 'pathological jealousy' and the defence gave a detailed history of his mental health problems. Unsurprisingly, because of these problems, he was found guilty of manslaughter rather than murder. The judge sentenced him to six years. I do not know how many he served.

Mark's failure to connect with the facts of his crime, plus his psychological state when he committed it, are, it seems to me, characteristic of middle-aged marital homicide. For it is at this junction in life, its midpoint, when husbands and wives are most likely to kill each other. Sometimes, both will die at the same time: one murder, one suicide. In later life, concurrent deaths often have a different cause but, at this stage, murder-suicide is the likely explanation when two bodies are found. And, indeed, Mark came close to killing himself as well as Zoe. He inflicted three deep stab wounds on his own body and was hospitalized for twelve days. I would say that in the majority of intended murder-suicides the killer fails to complete the plan and kill him or herself, although there are some startling exceptions.

Murder and manslaughter are both homicide: the exact charge depends on the intention of the perpetrator, and disentangling these intentions inside a marriage, where emotions constantly ebb and flow, can be a difficult job for the Crown Prosecution Service and, ultimately, the jury.

I was called to another mortuary one drizzly afternoon to carry out a post-mortem on a man who had been mugged in the street. Robert Cargill was of short stature and so painfully thin that his face was like a skull. A mop of black hair curled around his temples but now this was soaked in blood.

An officer identified him formally and gave his age as forty-five.

'Was he found in the road?' I asked the police officers as the smell of alcohol wafted out from the body to every corner of the post-mortem room.

'Nope, at home in his living room,' they said.

I raised my eyebrows.

'How on earth did he get in there?'

'Wife said that she went out to look for him and found him lying face down in a hedge. He managed to stagger home with her supporting him. She lay him down on the floor and he said he thought he'd be all right. She went to bed, woke up later and he was dead.'

Looking at the man's injuries, I was incredulous.

'Why didn't she call an ambulance?' I asked.

The officers exchanged glances.

'She's known to us,' they said. 'She's a bit of a drunk.'

'She couldn't even dial 999? Wasn't there anyone else around to do it?'

They shrugged.

'There's a child,' said one. 'But he's only six.'

'Did she show you the hedge?'

'Yeah, it's a couple of houses down the road.'

'But just look at him!' A glance told me that here was a badly fractured skull. And his face had taken such a bloody beating that I was sure no human fist could have caused the damage. His assailant must have had a heavy, metal weapon.

'Are there signs of a struggle on the pavement or in the hedge?' I asked.

They shook their heads. So they probably did not believe the woman's story either, but were waiting for me to corroborate their doubts.

It didn't take long. For a start, hypostasis, that tell-tale marker by red blood cells of a body's position after death, indicated that he had died sitting down and had remained that way for some time afterwards. As for his injuries, I could not see how it was possible for him to have walked in off the street, even with his wife's help. I found that beneath the facial bruises and lacerations were extensive fractures; of the left side of the skull, the left cheekbone and the left jaw.

The brain was bruised and bloody from sub-arachnoid haemorrhages. The hands were badly bruised and I was pretty sure that was because he had been trying ineffectively to defend himself.

'Well?' asked the officers when I had finished.

'I think he was hit while he was drunk and fairly incapable. You can smell him and you've seen his liver. I'm sure that tox will reveal a very high alcohol level. The weapon used has left a clear impression here . . . If I had to guess what it was, I'd say a round-headed hammer. It was used repeatedly and with force. There is no way he could have got up and walked in off the street with these injuries.'

'So . . . you think he was killed in his own house?' they asked.

I nodded.

'While he was sitting in a chair. I don't know how she got him on the floor afterwards, but this injury around the left ear is different. It looks to me as if, once he was down, someone stamped on his face.'

They did not speak.

'Was there evidence that anyone else was home?' I asked. 'Apart from the child?'

There was a silence.

'No,' said the senior investigating officer at last.

They said that they would contact me when they had talked to Mrs Cargill again. In fact, they sent me a transcript of her confession.

'The money I was earning was just enough to cover the mortgage. But when Bobby lost his job through drinking, I had to use the mortgage money to buy food for the family. Bobby found work at Mulligans, but then one day I came home and found a Mulligans van outside. He'd been on the drink again and they'd given him lots of chances so now I knew that the van meant he'd lost his job. It was outside for a few days. When the man came from Mulligans, Bobby wouldn't give him the keys so eventually they towed it away.

'I very often had to borrow money from the man across the road; he was very nice. And Bobby's mother gave us money, too, and his brother loaned us some. But Bobby wasn't working and I began to get desperate as the bills came in and we couldn't pay them. I was afraid to open the envelopes. I changed jobs and became a cleaner because then I could do lots of overtime.

'I noticed that the odd note would disappear from my purse, but Bobby always denied taking it. He was drinking a lot and betting a bit as well. Then he got a sort of on-off job with a haulage contractor. I was earning good overtime now and Bobby brought some in, but when he was off on the drink he didn't earn anything and this lasted for weeks at a time. One Saturday I tried to go shopping and found that £100 was missing from my purse. When I asked Bobby about it, he denied taking it and said my sisters had taken it. One of them came round and confronted him, and then he confessed: he said he'd had a tip on a horse that had gone down. But after that I knew I couldn't trust him.

'He has been violent on a number of occasions. About a year ago he said he was going to tip hot fat over me from the chip pan. And, a few times, he tried to strangle me and, once, I did push our son in front of me because I knew he would not hit a child. I called the police and they warned him off; otherwise, I kept my troubles to myself. I did not see a doctor about my injuries.

'One or two Saturdays ago we didn't have any money. He asked me to steal him some drink. I took some vodka and some meat at Sainsbury's – but I was caught. When I was arrested, I was in a state of shock. I didn't really struggle. By now we hadn't paid the mortgage for over a year. The bank took us to court, I went, but the case was delayed. His mother sent some money to help with the bills, but he took it for drink, even though the gas had been cut off. At the moment I am still working as a cleaner. Bobby lost his job at the haulage company after he was arrested for drunk driving.

'This Saturday he said he was going out for some cigarettes at four in the afternoon. He did not reappear until ten thirty at night. When he came in, I was in the living room. He went into the kitchen first and then came into the living room. I asked him where he had been. He didn't answer me. He was staggering. He put his keys on the mantelpiece and sat down in the armchair, half doped and half asleep.

'I was sure that he had brought some other drink with him. He often hides drink, and I have also found his empty bottles on the top of cupboards or under the bed. I looked in the kitchen but did not find any on Saturday. But I remember seeing the hammer in the kitchen cupboard. I remember picking it up. I was taking antibiotics for a dog bite and it must have been the pills, because I wouldn't harm anyone. I am so sad, because I loved him. He never worked much. I never meant to kill him, though.

'I was in front of him in the living room with the hammer, shouting at him. I don't remember hitting him a lot of times. I don't remember seeing any blood. I think I fell asleep, and when I woke up I thought he was asleep, too, but when I went to feel him I knew he was dead. I didn't know what to do or where to turn. There was a lot of blood about. I set about cleaning it up. It was on the curtains, too, and I washed them and hung them on the line in the garden. The hammer was beside him. I put it back in the kitchen cupboard but then took it out again and washed it and put it in a carrier bag. I put it down the garden in the shed. I put my clothes in a plastic bucket and left that outside by the washing line. I moved him so he was lying on the floor, and I could only just get him out of the chair, he was so heavy.

'I walked down the road but then had second thoughts and went back and did more cleaning up. I thought I would have to face someone sooner or later. But I didn't do anything. My mind was not right.

'Finally, I phoned my sister and she phoned the police and I told them all lies. I said that I'd found Bobby in a hedge and that he'd been mugged.'

Ongoing questioning revealed that the wife had left something important out of her story. That was her own alcohol consumption. She was described by friends and family, as well as the police, as, like her husband, a very heavy drinker. Her own statement said: 'I am not an alcoholic, but I felt that he was driving me to it. I have been drinking more recently than normally.'

At least part of her fury turned out under further questioning to be not her husband's unexplained absence that Saturday afternoon but his arrival at home apparently without any drink for her. More specifically, she believed he had deliberately hidden a full bottle in the kitchen on his return so that she would not find it. She was right. He had brought vodka, which he hid high on a cupboard before falling asleep in the armchair. She searched the kitchen in vain and now, added to the long years of marital suffering, was the feeling that he had cheated her out of a drink. It was the last straw. On finding no bottle, she had grabbed the hammer.

It is interesting that she fell asleep after killing him. She had certainly been drinking earlier in the day, but perhaps she slept now from a sense of relief – because she did know that he was dead and she understood that the pain and worry Bobby had caused her were over. After waking and clearing up, but before phoning the police, she found the missing bottle and drank a large proportion of it.

When the police arrived, the officer remembered her from the shoplifting incident the week before and greeted her by name. He received little response. He said: 'She was drunk, unsteady on her feet and her eyes were glazed. [In order to arrest her . . .] I had to assist her to step over the body. But she was so unsteady that the heel of her right shoe caught the forehead of the deceased.'

This officer's statement was sent to me with the question: could this account for the stamping injury you found on Bobby Cargill's face?

I said it probably could.

Many people will understand, even if they cannot condone, the actions of Mrs Cargill. Her allegations of Bobby's violence were substantiated by family and neighbours. This abuse, and her struggles to feed the family while he consistently drank away all the money she earned, would be problematic enough for a capable and educated woman who understood the legal system: there was little chance that this wife, struggling in low-paid work, would use the police and legal means to protect herself from a husband she evidently could not contemplate leaving.

And would the law anyway have protected her? In about 40 per cent of homicides where the victim is female, the partner or ex-partner is suspected. The homicide very often follows a long marital history of abuse, domestic violence, police intervention and court orders. There are even cases of men returning home and murdering their spouse when released on bail after being charged with assaulting her.

When a man kills a partner, male or female, in my experience it is usually a response to a threat or intention to leave. No one accused Mark of abuse before he killed Zoe, but his insistence that his motivation was love (saying that now they would be together in death) is typical of many of the domestic homicides which are about retaining control over a partner who threatens to start a new life. Mark deluded himself that by killing Zoe he could stop her leaving and somehow freeze their marriage. This is one crime where the perpetrator nearly always presents himself as a victim.

Abusers kill, but so do the abused – and although this is certainly a response to brutality, it is seldom an act of self-defence. It generally follows years of domestic violence and/or living with an intolerable degree of coercive control (controlling, non-violent behaviour was made an offence in 2015); in my files, this is the most likely back story when a woman murders a man. And it is rare. While male partners are usually the first suspect in a murder investigation, female partners are suspected in only 4 per cent of male homicides.

I would be amazed, in Mrs Cargill's case, and many others, if she had not often daydreamed about the release her husband's death might bring her. From daydreaming about a natural death, it is both a very large and a very small step to bringing about the longed-for release by actually causing that death. The action may apparently come from nowhere – nearly all statements contain phrases like this wife's insistence that she was not the kind of person to kill someone, that the antibiotics she was taking had made her behave uncharacteristically, that she loved the deceased – but the reality may be that fury, alcohol, pain, long-term suffering, or all four, trigger a loss of control which at some unacknowledged level has long been a fantasy. This greatly complicates intent and, until law reforms in 2010 which recognized the pressure of living with long-term domestic violence, the abused who turned on their abuser tended to face murder rather than manslaughter charges. Mrs Cargill did not. Her repeated hammer blows supported her case that this was a sudden, momentary, extreme loss of control rather than the result of any calculation and she received a short sentence for manslaughter.

I will take you just once more into the dark labyrinth of fatal midlife marital difficulties before I suggest why a woman married to that well-off and well-respected judge, described by Shakespeare as being, in midlife, *full of wise saws and modern instances*, might not have shared the world's admiration for him but actually have wanted to murder her husband.

I 2

We sat with our cups of tea in the mortuary, examining a collection of pictures.

'Deceased lived here . . .' the junior detective said, passing around a photo of a large and respectable Victorian town house. It was very clean, with all surfaces bare. There was modern, quite expensive furniture.

'How many kids?' his colleague asked.

'Two.' He handed us pictures of bedrooms that were a great deal less tidy than the rest of the house. The floor of each was covered in discarded clothes and criss-crossed by wires and gadgets.

'Teenagers,' he explained, unnecessarily.

It was December, a time of good will for some and murder for others. There was a tree in the living room and Christmas cards were neatly arranged in a vertical holder. In the kitchen, someone had been systematically writing their way through a list of cards to send. The box was open on the table. Each card barked: 'Peace at Christmastime!' Completed envelopes, stamped, had been stacked neatly to one side.

This was an entirely normal family house in December, except that it was covered in blood. In the bathroom, the kitchen, the living room, the hallway. Almost every door handle was smeared red, there were towels soaked in blood on the landing and on the stairs, and the bathroom floor was covered by a large, red puddle.

'Why isn't Daniel's body in the pictures?' I asked. 'Did the paramedics think they could save him?'

'The paramedics got there first and the doctor was right behind them in a helicopter. Said he'd operate then and there.'

'On the bathroom floor?'

'Yep.'

Brave doctor.

'They thought he'd saved Daniel. The nearest trauma hospital was quite close, so they got him in the wagon, but he went straight downhill. Died a few minutes later, pretty much at the entrance to A&E.'

'What's the wife saying?' asked the senior officer.

'Nothing.'

The officer raised his eyebrows.

'But apparently, when the paramedics got there, she opened the door and was still holding the knife.'

'Where is she?'

'At the station. She's barely said a word.'

'Shock,' the senior detective said wisely.

'Not as shocked as the husband, though.' The coroner's officer put down his mug and stood up.

'Amazing how often people kill someone else then go into shock themselves,' another officer said as we trooped off to change.

'Just as well,' the boss agreed. 'They're much easier to arrest.'

Daniel lay waiting for us in the post-mortem room. He was forty-five, not tall, but slim and strong. His face was gaunt and a few deep lines were chiselled around his eyes and mouth in places that would have been smooth a few years ago. There were flecks of grey in his dark, curly hair and, at his temples, white hairs were winning their battle against the black ones.

There was evidence of the strenuous attempts to save Daniel. An endotracheal tube was still *in situ*, he had numerous intravenous injection sites but, most noticeably of all, there was a large surgical incision right across his chest, an incision called a clam shell, loosely sutured with large stitches.

The stab wounds were immediately obvious, and they were all on the front of his body. One was adjacent to the left nipple; another was very nearby. They looked deep. A third was about a centimetre away, but it was so superficial it had barely broken the skin. And there was another, similarly superficial, horizontal injury across the left wrist. When I turned the body over, I found a complex group of rather strange abrasions on the back of his left shoulder.

Daniel had taken good care of himself. His hair was trimmed and showed no signs of thinning and, from his muscle tone, it seemed he had maintained a good level of physical fitness. But his body, like every body, would have peaked at around twenty-five. The slow, inevitable decline of senescence had been underway for twenty years. For twenty years, irreplaceable cells had been dying.

Some cells in our bodies do regenerate throughout life, but even this ability can diminish over time. Many cells are simply lost. Most importantly, the heart does not regenerate cells. Neither does most of the brain. Neither do some of the important bits of the kidneys. The compensation is this: we have a bit more heart, quite a lot more brain and substantially more kidney than perhaps we really need. The excess gives us a little resilience against ageing. But age we must.

We know that exposure to sunlight can make the skin less elastic. Skin cells do regenerate, and they can do a lot of repair work, but one long-term result of this exposure is certainly wrinkles. However, two people can be exposed to exactly the same amount of sunlight over a number of years and one will have wrinkled skin by the age of forty and the other not until the age of eighty. The difference, of course, lies in the genes. And if that can happen outside the body, it is safe to assume that something similar is going on inside us, controlling the rate at which various cells die. Our own individual ageing timeline must be genetically determined – but our environment and lifestyle can impact greatly on that pre-determination.

Daniel, like most of us, would probably have claimed that there was no noticeable effect of the ageing process on his body. He might have said that, at forty-five, he felt exactly the same as he had at twenty-five. There was, however, a thin build-up of fat around his abdomen which I expect had been less noticeable and more evenly distributed ten years ago. He may already have needed glasses to read or was wondering if he ought to have his eyes tested. Since he kept physically fit, a toll of small injuries may have left some damage. And, if pushed, he might have agreed that he had received treatment for minor ailments that were more persistent than he had expected. Or he might privately have admitted to some worries about his digestion or an increasing amount of dental work.

None of this will have impacted significantly on his life. And, pathologically, most of the evidence of his ageing was at a microscopic level. For instance, the kidneys have a complex and ingenious filtering process that keeps what we need in our blood supply and gets rid of toxins and excess chemicals. Blood is pushed through tiny bunches of filtering capillaries known as glomeruli. In Daniel, as in most forty-five-year-olds, some of these glomeruli were missing. There might have been an infection in the past, now long forgotten, or the kidneys could have been exposed to environmental toxins, unwillingly or willingly consumed (any area of the body involved in waste disposal can suffer from exposure to alcohol, nicotine and other substances our brains tell us we enjoy), but by this age the kidney filtration system is, in a few sporadic places, simply absent.

When I examined Daniel's heart, I found a sure indicator of age: lipofuscin, a delightful, glittery pigment that cells don't want or need but which they cannot eliminate. In some circumstances its accumulation causes problems (it can play a role in macular degeneration of the eye) but generally this microscopically gorgeous and pathologically pretty waste product builds up harmlessly in various organs over the years. The amount of lipofuscin can give a fairly accurate indication of age, just as archaeologists might assess how long a site was once occupied from the size of its rubbish heaps. At Daniel's age, it was liberally scattered, as if tiny, shiny confetti had been blown across his heart by the wind.

Had he been aware of any of these microscopic changes? Of course not. Had he been aware of the heart valve problem I found? Probably not. When his notes arrived from his GP there was no mention of it. Although it was not the reason he was here and had not played a direct role in his death, it was, nevertheless, something significant I had to point out in his post-mortem report.

We have four heart valves, each a gatekeeper to a different chamber or vessel of that amazing organ, each a remarkable feat of engineering in itself. They work in concert to direct the blood and make sure it doesn't flow backwards. The heart valves are so diaphanous that you can put a finger on one side and see at least the colour of that finger from the other.

They are only about an inch in diameter, made from a thin connective tissue which is designed perfectly for the job. And that job is to be both robust and flexible enough to snap open and then closed, folding and collapsing again and again, as pressure falls and rises, seventy times a minute, for as long as a hundred years. And if you want to know how great that pressure is, rising suddenly and sharply hundreds of millions of times over a life before falling again, just stand by the sea during a gale. Yes, heart valves are truly extraordinary.

The left side of the heart has a harder job to do and takes the most pressure: it receives oxygenated blood from the lungs and the valves help force it into the body's main artery to begin its circular journey. The first valve the blood flows through on its voyage, the mitral valve, is subject to the greatest pressure changes. But the second, the aortic valve, must also be very tough. If there are valve problems, it is usually in one of these two, sometimes both. On the other side of the heart, where deoxygenated blood is fed in from the major veins of the body – the vena cavae – on its way back to the lungs, the pressure is much lower and the valves are thinner and less prone to wear and tear.

For years, we only really knew about valve disease from studying the still organs of the dead. Now we know that the causes are various but, for a long time, when there was a mitral valve problem, one of the possible causes was assumed to have been an auto-immune response to rheumatic fever in childhood. Rheumatic fever is not unknown, even now, in the UK, but it is seldom encountered except in first-generation immigrants from less medically advanced parts of the world.

Prescribing antibiotics for sore throats brought about its decline here, although not soon enough for my mother, whose childhood in the 1920s pre-dated antibiotic use. I can therefore personally attest to the results of a seriously faulty mitral valve. In her case, this was caused by continuing inflammation of the heart valves after catching a bacterial infection that led to scarlet fever, years before as a girl.

She was in her late thirties when I was born and, during my childhood, she simply faded away, often not having sufficient energy to get up in the morning, or at least stay up once she'd seen me off to school. At her death, aged forty-seven, she had a post-mortem examination and, when I was at medical school, my father, shyly, gave me the report. It told me that her mitral valve had become far too thickened and stiff to open and close properly. Blood could not be pumped efficiently around her body.

Of course, this has given me a lifelong interest in heart valves and a huge respect for their hard work. The valves consist of two or three curved leaves, a shape I have been delighted to see replicated on fountains in Rome. The way they snap open and shut reminds me of a different culture entirely: that moment in all the best westerns when the bad guy bursts in through the saloon doors. They swing open for the blood to force its way through and then swing shut behind it. But now I looked hard at Daniel's saloon doors and I was sure they had lost their swing.

'This is interesting,' I said to the police officers. 'He had a faulty heart valve.'

The disappointment in the room was palpable.

'You're not going to tell me that's what killed him?' The senior detective was clearly alarmed.

'The wife had the knife in her hand!' repeated his junior.

'No, no, this isn't the cause of death,' I said. 'But it's still interesting.'

Looking at the impatient faces that surrounded me, I decided not to examine the heart valve further. Not just at the moment.

I had followed the track of the two significant injuries. One of them had passed upwards and to the left, missing the chest cavity completely and lodging about ten centimetres into the muscle of the chest wall. No doubt it had been very painful, but that had certainly not killed Daniel.

The other was just on the skin, a centimetre away, but it went in a different direction and had cut, fatally, into the front wall of the heart's left ventricle. More than that I could not tell because the doctor who had tried to save Daniel's life with his bathroom surgery had destroyed the track of the wound.

Emergency doctors, who arrive fast on wheels or even faster in a helicopter brilliantly piloted on to some small patch of land nearby, have to be ready to do anything at any time. But it's a brave doctor who rushes into a house and proceeds to open a patient's chest on the bathroom floor. And, given those circumstances, it's a churlish pathologist who begs and pleads with him to spare a thought next time for forensic evidence. However, this pathologist did phone the emergency doctor, whom I knew well, to ask him about the case and remind him of our different roles.

'Remember, it's not a dot-to-dot puzzle,' I said, and he laughed.

'Yeah, once I was inside his body, I realized I'd cut through the wound. Heat of the moment and it was a bloody small bathroom.'

It had been bloody, all right.

He knew as well as I that cutting just half a centimetre to one side and avoiding an obvious stab wound can make all the difference, should the patient die, to the understanding of a death forensically. And it won't alter the chances of successful surgery. Of course, the surgeon forgets this, driven by their intention that the patient will live. In this case, surgery had so nearly been successful: the wound to the heart was neatly sutured and, with some adrenaline, more blood transfusion and a lot of luck, it could have worked.

'I really thought I'd saved him,' the emergency doctor said mournfully. 'There was such a sudden improvement, but . . . well, anyway, we lost him again.'

The police officers moved in closer now to see the heart.

'You can see how the track of the knife has been decimated by the bathroom-floor surgery. Good doctoring if he'd lived, but it means I won't be able to give the degree of detail in my report that I'd like.'

'Heat of the moment,' they all agreed.

The senior detective added: 'Anyway, we don't need so much forensics, Doc. We've got the wife in custody. She'll soon confess.'

At that moment, his colleague, who had been taking a call, reappeared at my side.

'Wife's talking now,' he said. 'Says she didn't do it.'

'Don't tell me! She happened to be making dinner and he tripped and fell on the knife,' the coroner's officer scoffed. 'If I had a quid for every time someone's fallen on the knife . . . Allegedly.'

'You should hear what the neighbours had to say about her,' his colleague said.

I was surprised by this.

'What did the neighbours say?'

'They're one of those couples who don't fight when the kids are there. Then the kids go out and it all kicks off. She used to scream so loudly half the street could hear.'

I thought of the pictures of the teenagers' bedrooms, crammed with gaming hardware and hardly worn clothes. Do couples who stay together for the sake of their children really think the children believe that all is well?

'Not nice kids, not a nice wife,' the officer went on. 'Always shouting and swearing at Daniel here. Who never raised his voice, apparently.'

We all glanced at the motionless Daniel. Did he look as though he had been a quiet man? Passive, even? But his expressionless face revealed nothing.

'The kids shouted, too?' I asked.

'There are families in the houses on either side so . . . lots of witnesses. One bloke next door thinks the kids were terrible. Says that they were nicer to the dog than to their dad. Swearing, shouting at him. Then, when they were out, the mother used to start. By all accounts, she's a right bully. So, this morning the boys went off to spend the day with their grandparents, leaving Mummy and Daddy to wrap their humungous pile of Christmas presents. The neighbours knew as soon as the kids were out because the mother started yelling.'

'Local PC's notes say that he'd been overlooked for promotion,' the junior officer added.

'We all know how that feels,' one of his colleagues murmured.

'And,' continued the junior, 'we've got two – no, three – witnesses who heard her threatening to kill him.'

I raised my eyebrows.

'Really? Are you sure? What did she say?'

'Er . . .' He riffled through his notes. '"I'd like to kill you." The other witness says it was: "I want to kill you." And a lady next door on the left thinks she heard "I'm going to kill you."'

'And what's the wife's story?' I asked.

'She's saying he stabbed himself.'

There was some more scoffing, and the junior officer gave a hollow laugh I suspected he'd learned from his elders at the police station.

'Actually,' I said, 'I think it's most likely that he did.'

It was one of those moments when all the officers in the room turn to you with a mixture of disappointment and disbelief bordering on incredulity because you've said exactly what they don't want to hear.

The coroner's officer almost laughed.

'Stabbed himself? With his wife standing watching?'

'Nah,' the senior detective said. 'If you're going to stab yourself, you don't do it while your wife's writing Christmas cards.'

I looked back at them. 'It seems to me that all his injuries are self-inflicted.'

'Come on, Doc.'

'But she wouldn't just stand there and watch, would she?'

'The children aren't at home,' I said. 'And so the parents start on each other. They get very angry and she says that she wants to kill him. He says something like: "Go on, then!"'

'Calling her bluff?'

'Or perhaps he really thought he wanted to die. Maybe she fetched the knife, but maybe he even got it for her.'

The kitchen knife was sitting nearby, tightly sealed in an evidence box with a plastic window so you could see but not touch it. The blade was smeared with blood. I was sure it was the right knife.

'Then, possibly he handed it to her. And said something like: "You want to kill me. Do it, then." And she said –'

The officer who had been on the phone interrupted me.

225

'Actually . . . actually, according to the statement she's just given, she fetched the knife. And he said: "I'd rather be dead than carry on like this."'

'And according to her, what did she say?'

'"Don't do it." Says she pleaded with him.'

The junior detective was looking through his witness notes.

'No one actually heard any pleading . . .' he said. 'From what the neighbours told us, I thought he must have had the knife and been threatening her. I thought she was going to say there was a struggle for the knife and when she got hold of it she used it in self-defence.'

'Nope,' said the officer who had taken the phone call. 'That's not her story.'

The junior detective shuffled through a few pages and then read: 'Right, this is what the neighbours heard. "Go on, go on, get on with it, go on." One bloke thinks that she also said: "Do it for me!" but another lot heard: "Do your children a favour!"'

He looked from face to face and there was a long silence. My job takes me to the murkiest places in the human soul, but I find few things more troubling than the crowds who jeer, shout, goad and cajole hesitant, anguished people in high places until they leap to their deaths. If the neighbours were to be believed, it now began to seem that this wife had done something similar to Daniel. I thought about the anger, the hurt, the spite, the disappointment, the history, the years of unhappiness, which had fuelled this final challenge. Of course, the couple were over forty. That's how long it takes to create such a mess.

'What makes you so sure he did it himself, Doc?' the coroner's officer asked.

'These are all pretty much classic wounds of self-infliction, and that superficial wound across the left wrist is a red flag. I mean, if Daniel had been attacked with a knife, his wrist might just possibly have been slashed – but not horizontally like that.'

We all stared at his body in silence. 'It's impossible to look at the wounds and be sure about the order of events,' I said. 'But I could have a guess.'

Many detectives don't like pathologists to play Sherlock Holmes. They think making deductions is their job, not mine. So even on the occasions when I am quite confident that I know what happened, there are police officers who really don't want to hear it. If only they knew that Conan Doyle had based his investigator on a doctor and not on a policeman. However, these officers were curious. They even joined in.

'Bet the wrist was first,' one said.

I agreed.

And the junior officer said: 'It's obvious that the last thing to happen was the stab wound which killed him.'

I shook my head. 'Not necessarily. Because it wouldn't have killed him instantly. Once the wife had challenged him to kill himself, he tried the wrist and realized how hard that was going to be and perhaps how . . . undramatic. He's giving her what she says she wants now, but he'd like her to suffer. So he rips open his shirt and sticks the knife in his chest and it goes straight into his heart. For a moment there is nothing. Then she panics when she sees a gush of blood. She grabs a towel and tries to mop it up. He pushes her off and staggers around the house with her supplying towels and him dropping them and, between them, they get blood everywhere.

'By now, Daniel probably thinks he should be dead. But he isn't, so he assumes he's missed his heart. Determined to finish the job off, he sticks the knife in again. More panic, more towels . . . when he collapses on the bathroom floor, she's still mopping up blood. But actually, the second wound only went into the chest wall. He'd been successful first time around, he just didn't know it. She calls the ambulance . . . do we know what she said?'

One of the officers consulted his notes. 'Erm . . . she said: "My husband's got a knife in his chest and he's bleeding to death."'

The senior detective looked thoughtful. 'Doesn't say he stuck it in himself.'

The younger detective said: 'Well, if the doc's right, I mean, if the neighbours heard her goading him into doing it, she as good as stuck it in him.'

'Not in law,' his boss told him.

The coroner's officer asked: 'Doc, how long does it take to die when you've got a knife in your heart?'

I shrugged.

'Depends exactly where the knife goes in. A lot of people crumple and die quite quickly on the spot, but some of them manage to run a hundred yards. A wound like that in the left ventricle doesn't necessarily kill you instantly because it takes a while for blood to escape, pressure to drop, circulation to fall away and the heart to lose its battle against the leak. He might be expected to miss his heart with the second stab because I doubt he was feeling too well by then.'

'How sure are you of all this?' the senior detective asked. 'I mean, how do you know Daniel didn't start with the wrist and then stop? And then, she took the knife and stuck it in him?'

I thought about that. I have colleagues who are always sure. Is their certainty a function of character or youth? Even when young, I could never be a hundred per cent sure of anything. There were always options, variable factors and different views to consider. And I can't even be dogmatic now. My experience of life's inconsistencies and surprises, its twists, coincidences and contradictions, always leaves total certainty out of my reach. So often, in court, I have had to admit that some extreme scenario suggested in all serious-ness by a confident barrister might *just*, well, in theory, be possible. Then, somehow, I have to make sure the jury knows that it's an outside, lottery chance.

'Of course, I can never be absolutely sure,' I said. 'I can only say that's what I see in these wounds. First, because the sites are all reachable. Second, because the track of a self-inflicted chest stab by a right-handed person usually goes up and to the left, as both of these wounds do. And I can say the cut across the left wrist is indicative of that intention – it is so minimal that it is most unlikely to have been the last wound. But, no, I can't entirely rule out the possibility that the wife took the knife and stabbed him.'

'What about those strange marks on his back?' the junior detective asked.

'Nothing suspicious there. When he fell, he fell against something, that's all. I can soon work out what from the pictures.'

There was a long silence.

'I want to charge her,' the senior detective concluded. 'If she goaded Daniel into doing it, she came as close as she could to stabbing him without actually touching the knife. And if the doc says there's a possibility that she *did* take the knife . . .'

The detectives left the post-mortem room still discussing this. They had all the information they needed now. I stayed behind with the mortuary assistants and the photographer to do some more dissection.

Now I could look closely at Daniel's heart, particularly its mitral valve. The other valves have three leaves, the mitral has two, perhaps to give it the extra strength it needs to sustain a lifetime of such intense pressure changes. I had already removed the heli-med doctor's sutures to examine the stab wound and now this made close examination of the valve easier.

However, nothing seemed to be wrong with either the leaflets of the valve or the tiny guy ropes which fasten it to the muscle. They look very like the cords that attach a skydiver to their billowing parachute. Here, they were all intact. So the problem was not obvious, although its effects were clear.

The left atrium is said to be the heart's first chamber. It is designated as the starting point of the blood's circumnavigation of the body. It holds the blood which has been oxygenated by the lungs and then, when full, pumps it through the mitral valve into the next chamber: the left ventricle. From here it is forced into the main artery for its journey around the body. I was sure that the inside wall of Daniel's left atrium was not normal. There was a white patch in it, a small area of thickened tissue.

This is called a jet lesion, and it is damage caused by blood leaking backwards through a floppy mitral valve.

I decided to try an experiment in the sink. I put the heart under the tap so that the water flowed into the ventricle from the aorta – in other words, in the opposite direction from the usual blood flow. I put my finger over the stab wound so that the heart was leakproof again and watched as the left ventricle filled. A full ventricle: that's what builds up the pressure to help push the blood on its journey. But, in Daniel's case, it meant that the mitral valve was bulging suspiciously upwards into the atrium until . . . whoosh. A jet of water flew into the wall of the atrium exactly where it was white and thickened. Yes. A positive diagnosis. A tiny stream of blood had been hitting that wall through a gap between the two edges of the mitral valve for years. Because, although this condition can certainly be caused, like my mother's, by infection – the heart valves are notorious traps for bacteria – Daniel had been born in the UK in the era of antibiotics. In him, the problem was much more likely to be congenital.

Many people with mitral valve faults have no symptoms throughout their life and die from different causes. But this jet lesion would soon have required attention. It could have only got worse and it was already sufficiently pronounced for me to suspect that Daniel had an inkling of his heart problem.

Sure enough, when I was sent his wife's statement, I read that he had been very upset at recent palpitations in his chest. His father had died at the age Daniel had now reached, forty-five, from an unidentified heart problem. Daniel, it seemed, had been increasingly concerned by his own symptoms, so concerned that, instead of visiting his doctor, he had stayed away in fear. If only he had made that appointment. My mother's open-heart surgery was pioneering in the early 1950s, but there were no artificial valves then. Now there are, and I'm sure she would have benefited from this advance if she had lived just a few years longer.

So here was a man under a lot of stress with deep-seated medical worries he was scared to address and an ominous sense that, like his father at forty-five, his own death was imminent. Recent lack of success at work, a home which was far from peaceful and some difficult family relationships were all becoming increasingly hard to manage. All this added up to the psychological precursors of a suicide.

The neighbours certainly blamed his wife for goading him, but she could only have been successful if he had been predisposed to killing himself. Some suicides are calculated to make those who have inflicted pain experience pain themselves. I don't know if that was the case here. I don't know if remorse might be appropriate for her to feel, nor if she did so. After much deliberation with the Crown Prosecution Service, the police decided not to charge her.

At Daniel's inquest, she was the archetypal grieving widow who was treated with kid gloves – by everyone but the coroner, that is, because she point-blank refused to give verbal evidence about the events of that day.

A verdict of suicide is one of the few that must be reached on the higher level of proof – beyond reasonable doubt. The coroner concluded that this degree of proof had not been reached. He returned an open verdict.

13

Looking at a map of tectonic plates recently, I began to understand how a large earthquake may be caused by small movements in loosely connected, faraway fault lines. I suspect that the reason so many lives and marriages fall apart in early middle age can be similarly traced.

By the age of forty most of us have left freedom from responsibility behind. And illness, bereavement, bankruptcy, house moves, divorce, redundancy and other strains do not occur in isolation now. They are linked to a network of stress fractures, like difficult teenage children, elderly parents, limited job prospects, marital strain, debt. Our actions in the first half of our lives are often fuelled by our expectations for the future. Now the future is here. And it may be disappointingly different from the one we have imagined.

When I reached this stage in life, the pressures were relieved by learning to fly. I finally stopped looking up at aeroplanes and started looking out of their front windows instead. The responsibilities of my job and growing family were significant, but they meant that I could now find and fund an hour a week, just one amazing hour, to escape. Looking back, I realize that a small part of me lived for those Friday afternoons. It is hard to describe how exciting they were. The study, the preparation, the concentration. And then the wheels stopped rattling on the runway, the nose pointed upwards and there followed that extraordinary moment of silence at the junction between land and air. An instant of infinite promise. A heartbeat missed, a breath held, and I knew that I was no longer on this earth but rising above it.

Space opened around me. I had been entirely enclosed all week and hadn't even realized it, not until all the walls began to disappear. The view grew bigger and bigger and then it became a horizon. It was curved like something perfectly engineered. I could sense its infinity. And I was surrounded by absolutely nothing but air and a few clouds, wafting past like friendly neighbours. What a vast, beautiful, wonderful place the world seemed from up there. How benign it was. Life's tedious detail grew smaller as I flew higher until it was all reduced to nothingness. What did I think about? Nothing! Apart from flying the plane, of course. The dead – their bodies, their secrets – were far away.

All too soon, the demands of earthly existence extinguished my Friday hour. The absence of flying was keenly felt and lasted for some years. Then, finally, I was back in a plane again. I felt the same joy at returning to this layer of the earth's atmosphere that astronauts must feel as they arrive back from the opposite direction. When my fault lines did snap, much later in life, I wondered whether the quake might have struck earlier had it not been for my Friday-afternoon escapes, or if perhaps it might not have struck at all if I had flown more.

How do others dodge the critical pressures of midlife? Many attempt to alleviate pain by chemical means; death statistics reveal this, as they do so much about the way we live. I am referring particularly to the current record-breaking number of overdoses in this age group. In most cases, the fatal outcome is thought to be unintended, although some statistics show that a woman who dies through drug misuse is much more likely than a man to have caused her death deliberately.

The Office for National Statistics notes a steep rise in the graphs relating to so-called generation X. They were introduced to narcotics by the raves that blossomed towards the end of the twentieth century. We suspect that the habits formed then, resulting in serious subsequent drug use or dependency, is taking its toll now that this generation is at midlife and their bodies are losing some resilience. More than half of these deaths are, as ever, caused by opiates, but cocaine deaths doubled between 2015 and 2018. The only area of drug death decline is in those caused by paracetamol, which may simply be due to stricter controls on its sale since 1988.

And that other route to oblivion, my own drug of choice? Although alcohol-related deaths peak a little later in life, it is worth noting that they are seven times higher in the forty to forty-four age group in the UK than the average across all ages.

It seems that many of us have tied ourselves in knots by the time we reach our forties, and we face the choice of continuing as we are while the knots tighten, or loosening and retying them, or cutting them completely. While suicide is a very significant cause of death – indeed, it peaks at this age – another phenomenon starts to appear.

I was called to a small cottage where a man was half lying on the kitchen floor, his hip wedged against a table leg, the top half of his body, face down, against a bench. There were cushions beneath his face that were soaked in blood and the left side of his forehead was caked with it as far as his eye. It had run down his cheeks in places. Despite the mess, it was immediately clear that there was a single wound to the left temple. Car keys and an overflowing ashtray sat on a nearby table, as well as a plastic bottle with a pipe inserted on one side, aluminium cans, many lighters . . . unmistakably, drugs paraphernalia. Beneath all this, on the floor by the deceased's left hand was a Colt revolver.

The forensic firearms specialist joined me as I examined the scene and, leaving the police to establish whether the deceased was left-handed, we followed the body to the nearest mortuary. Here, under bright lights, surveyed by a very large police team, we cleaned up the wound. Now we could see that the bullet had entered in the middle of the temple. The hole was about 0.5 cm in diameter and surrounded by soot, which was dotted in an oval for about 2 cm around the wound.

This peppering was dense at the centre but sparser at its outer edges, which indicated that firing had been at close range. When a weapon has actually been in contact with the skin, the hot gases and smoke that follow the bullet out of the muzzle raise a ragged dome of skin that is radially split by the pressure. That was not the case here.

The trajectory of the bullet had been upwards into the head and through the man's brain. It had impacted in the centre of the top of the skull, an irregular fracture radiating from it.

The police were keen to press charges. They had arrested his ex-partner, who had presented herself some five hours after the body had been found. She had been visiting when, she claimed, he had produced the revolver, held it to his head and pulled the trigger. Nothing had happened. There had been a terrible pause while they both realized the gun had not gone off and he was still alive. He had then laughed and explained that he was playing Russian roulette. She said that she had immediately tried to wrestle the revolver from him but he had shaken her off, put the gun back to his head and pulled the trigger a second time.

The police did ask the partner if the deceased was left- or

right-handed. She replied without hesitation that he was left-handed. They arrested her anyway.

Russian roulette has cropped up at irregular intervals in my career. The deceased is always male, nearly always aged between forty and fifty and wishing to demonstrate a disregard for life which he may or may not truly feel. I wouldn't say this deadly game is prompted by suicidal feelings so much as a sense of pointlessness. The thinking usually is: well, if I don't die, I must be here for a reason. There must be a point. And if I do die . . . I won't know anything about it, will I? Readers may recognize the role alcohol or drugs might well play in this devil-may-care thinking. So I awaited the toxicology in this case with interest.

It revealed that the deceased had consumed no alcohol. He was slim and appeared reasonably fit and certainly showed no overt signs of being an addict. But his home was full of rubbish and drug paraphernalia and generally demonstrated the chaos I have learned to associate with addiction.

The toxicologist said that the deceased had smoked crack from the pipe on the table within two hours of his death, perhaps shortly before it, perhaps repeatedly. Crack produces a euphoria with which, I am told, whisky and soda simply cannot compete. The problem is that the euphoria doesn't last long and the misery of its come-down is legendary. Many users will do anything to ease that: mug or steal to buy more, or use other substances to soften the terrible blow. The most effective of these substances is heroin. But almost anything – Valium, alcohol, cannabis – is better than nothing to lessen the horror of the abyss.

The toxicologist thought that the deceased had done exactly that. He hadn't just smoked a lot of crack, he'd used a high dose of heroin to make himself feel better afterwards, as well as some cannabis. There is no question that he was under the influence of all three when Russian roulette started to seem like a good idea. I do wonder where he was in the pharmacological process of high, low, plateau. Was he still staring into the hideous crack abyss, in which case life had certainly become at least temporarily meaningless? Or had the heroin and cannabis taken hold and was he feeling warm, relaxed, cocooned . . . and safe? As if he could put a gun to his head and pull the trigger and nothing bad could possibly happen.

The police had become attached to the possibility that the former partner had shot him when he was incapacitated by crack or heroin, then cleared up the scene and invented the Russian roulette. Her clothes were immediately handed over to a gunshot residue forensic expert to see if her version of events could be corroborated.

He explains in his report that, when a cartridge is fired, the burning propellant produces residues in a cloud around the gun which are deposited on the skin and clothing of whoever fired the gun, as well as on persons and surfaces close by. Any handling or contact with a spent cartridge, recently fired weapon or contaminated surface can result in the transfer of those residues – but each leaves a different sort of pattern.

He found that the deceased had high levels of gunshot residue on both hands: primer residue, bullet residue and propellant. The amounts of both were about 50 per cent higher on the left hand than on the right. There was also residue on his clothing and the kitchen cupboards.

The ex-partner had no firearms residue or gun black on her hands or clothes but, as the police pointed out, there had been plenty of time for her to wash and change. The expert also said that, since primer residues take the form of very fine dust which is usually deposited within one or two metres of the discharge, most of it is lost from both hands and clothes within a few hours of firing.

His conclusion? There was no evidence that she had handled the gun at all and every reason to suppose that the deceased had done so with both hands. In fact, the expert concluded that the gun may have been fired when he was holding it not just with his left hand but with both.

What about the forensic scientist who arrived at the scene and specialized not in residues but in the firearms themselves?

He said that the .32 calibre Colt was rusty, in poor condition and not in proper working order. It was supposed to have both a single action and a double action, but it did not work at all in single-action mode. It worked in double action, but not correctly. Pulling back the trigger was supposed to rotate the cylinder so that each of the six chambers would align with the barrel in sequence. But when the expert pulled the trigger, he found that the cylinder advanced by more than one chamber, or sometimes by not even one chamber, leaving the revolver misaligned for firing. Double-action firing required long, continuous 12-lb pressure on the trigger. However, he found the effort required for this revolver varied between 10 and 16 lb. One thing he was sure of: it could not have gone off by itself.

The land and groove marks on the bullets after test firing correlated with those on the one bullet that had killed the Russian-roulette player.

We don't know how much of a fighting chance he had given himself to win the game. In theory, one in six, the odds dropping to one in five the next time he pulled the trigger. But his was a faulty gun. And, although we know he died at the second attempt, we don't know how many times he had tried in the past. If this was really only the second time he had pulled the trigger, he had been unlucky. And certainly stupid.

The former partner was not charged and her story was accepted, despite the time lapse before she presented herself, her possible change of clothes, a few anomalies in her facts and the likelihood that she had cleared the scene of any evidence of her own drug use before the police arrived. At the inquest, the coroner was convinced that this had been a deliberate act and that, despite the drugs, the deceased believed that the shot would kill him. She gave a verdict of suicide.

She was, I am sure, correct. But for me this death was more complicated than that. I think it was a halfway house between here and suicide: the let's-see-if-I-live-or-die that is characteristic of people at midlife who are not entirely sure that they want to carry on and not entirely sure that they don't.

Actual suicide perhaps carries a stronger sense of conviction. It is a leading cause of death for middle-aged women, but breast cancer is more than twice as likely to kill a woman than she is to kill herself. For men in midlife, suicide tops the fatality chart, along with overdose. Halfway through life, perhaps some people look back with pain and forward without hope. And so the decision is made not to continue.

I find suicides or half-suicides like this one particularly sad to investigate. I witness the acute suffering of friends and relatives and suspect that the deceased had no idea how much he or she really meant to those around them. Nor of how much they will be missed. Nor just how much their death would move the tectonic plates of the lives of those who knew them.

14

Here are some extracts from the statement of a woman describing her husband's behaviour prior to his death.

A. He was not good at holidays. He was always on call. He always had his mobile phone on . . . he became very much more taciturn. He became more difficult to talk to, he became more tense, withdrawn, and we as a family expressed this worry to each other.

Q. When can you date that from?

A. The last week of June, I would think . . . He was tired and looking his age. He seemed to have aged quite a bit. It is that last week in June particularly when we really noticed a great deal of change in him . . . He worried me somewhat one day, one evening, by suddenly getting up from his chair, having been quite withdrawn and worried, I think, and he went upstairs to dress, change his clothes. He came down looking rather smarter than he would normally be at home, rather smarter than he would normally be if he were just popping down to the local pub for a game of crib or something like that. He said he was going to [the pub] at the other end of the village, and off he went, seeming very preoccupied . . . About half an hour or 40 minutes later he came back, and I said: You have been quick . . . and he replied: I went for a walk instead to think something through. I was immediately worried, the way he said it. He said it slowly.

This man's crisis was precipitated by his work; he had found himself exposed to scrutiny and criticism which he felt tarnished his previously distinguished record. He believed he was unsupported by his employer. This lack of support added to a pre-existing feeling that he was undervalued; it followed a period of anomalies around his pension and his place in the pay structure.

His wife confirmed this under questioning.

Well, he often found that he was doing perhaps slightly lower-order jobs than he might be doing . . . when perhaps he might have been more involved in perhaps higher-level policy-making.

The man seems not to have shared his crisis with friends. Here his wife describes the nature of his friendships.

He always used to work so hard, because he was a work-aholic, to all intents, most of his friendships, in fact his close friendships, were all with people he worked with on a regular basis so, if he gave a regular briefing to someone, very often it would become not a close friendship but a friend-ship nevertheless.

His daughter reflected a sense of deepening crisis when she gave the following evidence about her father's behaviour before an important meeting.

He just seemed under an overwhelming amount of stress, that is the only way I can describe it, that there was some-thing on his mind. I would guess he was contemplating the next day, but he also seemed to be finding it almost painful to think about it. He was just very withdrawn, and I was just very, very concerned about him.

The man who was causing so much worry to his family was Dr David Kelly. I was not the pathologist who examined his body but was subsequently, in the light of widespread criticism of the way the case was conducted and even of the Hutton Inquiry (which controversially replaced an inquest into Dr Kelly's death), asked to review the case.

This suicide had both national and international repercussions and has been subjected to countless conspiracy theories. So I should first give some background into the details of the sad and extraordinary story.

The circumstances date from more than a decade before Dr Kelly's death. When Saddam Hussein, ruler of Iraq, invaded Kuwait in 1990, he was stopped by an international coalition and the United Nations sent inspectors to monitor his weapons-building programme. David Kelly, a UK expert in biological warfare, was one of those inspectors. He visited Iraq thirty-seven times in the seven years from the end of the First Gulf War until 1998.

By 1998, Hussein had started to repel the inspectors and there followed years of stand-offs, when the world tried to insist that Iraq's weaponry should be scrutinized and Iraq largely avoided this. The world took its information on Iraq's weapons-building from surveillance and secret intelligence sources. Secrecy, of course, can make reliability hard to assess. David Kelly continued to work for the British government, reviewing and interpreting information received from Iraq. It was part of his job to give off-the-record briefings to the press.

Suspected links between Iraq and the terrorists who had killed so many in New York on 11 September 2001 were probably a factor in the decision to invade the country early in the new century. But the overriding reason given was to stop Hussein's assumed weapons programme. This time there was not wide international support for military action; in fact, there were international protests against the possibility of war.

In March 2003, the USA, backed by a few allies, including the UK, but without United Nations approval, invaded Iraq. By 30 April, the invasion, but not the conflict, was over; Hussein had lost control of his country and the long-term socially, politically and militarily complex occupation of Iraq had begun.

The British government continued to insist that the invasion had been necessary. Their reasons had been stated clearly in a dossier they had produced the previous September, six months before the offensive. In his forward to it, Prime Minister Tony Blair had written:

> In recent months, I have been increasingly alarmed by the evidence from inside Iraq that, despite sanctions, despite the damage done to his capability in the past, despite the UN Security Council's Resolutions expressly outlawing it, and despite his denials, Saddam Hussein is continuing to develop Weapons of Mass Destruction and with them the ability to inflict real damage upon the region, and the stability of the world . . . his military planning allows for some of the WMD to be ready within 45 minutes of an order to use them.

On 22 May 2003, when the Iraq conflict was still dominant in the news headlines, Dr David Kelly agreed to give an off-the-record briefing to Andrew Gilligan, a BBC journalist. Gilligan was interviewed on the influential Radio 4 *Today* programme on 29 May, and said this about the September dossier and particularly the suggestion that Hussein could deploy weapons of mass destruction in just forty-five minutes:

Now that claim has come back to haunt Mr Blair because if the weapons had been that readily to hand, they probably would have been found by now. But you know, it could have been an honest mistake, but what I have been told is that the government knew that claim was questionable, even before the war, even before they wrote it in their dossier.

I have spoken to a British official who was involved in the preparation of the dossier, and he told me, until the week before it was published, the draft dossier produced by the Intelligence Services added little to what was already publicly known. He said: 'It was transformed in the week before it was published, to make it sexier. The classic example was the statement that weapons of mass destruction were ready for use within forty-five minutes. That information was not in the original draft. It was included in the dossier against our wishes, because it wasn't reliable. Most things in the dossier were double source, but that was single source, and we believed that the source was wrong.'

Now this official told us that the transformation of the dossier took place at the behest of Downing Street, and he added: 'Most people in intelligence weren't happy with the dossier, because it didn't reflect the considered view they were putting forward.'

This story challenged the legitimacy of the war and the integrity of the government. It received considerable publicity and created a furore between the government and the BBC. All this caused David Kelly increasingly acute discomfort as it became clearer and clearer that he was first *a* source of the story. Then, *the* source.

What did he actually say to Andrew Gilligan? Perhaps more than he meant to. Perhaps less than Gilligan suggested. We will never know; even the Hutton Inquiry, while openly critical of Gilligan, could not ascertain the exact truth. As a result of this BBC story, David Kelly was placed under a level of pressure he found unbearable. His employers decided, with little warning, to allow his exposure as the story's source, and there is no doubt that he believed himself utterly betrayed by them. Despite years of diligent service, he was publicly reprimanded and felt this belittled him. He was ordered to appear before two Parliamentary committees. In one, he felt himself to be questioned too rudely and aggressively. The whole session was televised, to his horror. It was an ordeal. A committee member even asked: '. . . *why did you feel it was incumbent upon you to go along with the request [to appear] that clearly had been made to you to be thrown to the wolves, not only to the media but, also, to this committee?'*

The very private workaholic found himself in the public glare, believing his job was in jeopardy and his life's work had been devalued. The Hutton Inquiry, set up to examine his death, may not always have agreed that David Kelly's feelings were justified. But it was those feelings which resulted in his suicide.

After his ordeal before the two parliamentary committees, David Kelly returned home. The next morning, the day of his death, he went to his study as usual (he worked primarily from home), as his wife recalled to the Hutton Inquiry.

Q. 17th July is a Thursday. What time did you get up that day?
A. About half past 8. It is rather later than normal.

246

Q. How did he seem?

A. Tired, subdued, but not depressed. I have no idea. He had never seemed depressed in all of this, but he was very tired and very subdued.

We now know that David Kelly had received an email that morning which contained a number of parliamentary questions. These were posed by Bernard Jenkin MP to the Secretary of State for Defence and basically called, in parliamentary language, for an investigation of David Kelly's meetings with Andrew Gilligan and for disciplinary action to be taken against the scientist. It must have been clear to Dr Kelly that this was a problem which was not going away and, indeed, it was escalating.

He had a quiet coffee break with his wife and then returned to his study. He wrote emails to the various colleagues who had sent messages of support, confirming that times were hard and saying how much he would like to get back to Iraq and get on with his job there. He did not stay at his desk for long. Janice Kelly confirmed this under questioning.

A. A few minutes later he went to sit in the sitting room all by himself without saying anything, which was quite unusual for him.

Q. . . . When was he sitting in the sitting room?

A. From about 12.30 I would think . . . he just sat and looked really very tired. By this time I had started with a huge headache and begun to feel sick. In fact I was physically sick several times at this stage because he looked so desperate.

Q. Did he have any lunch?

A. Yes, he did. I said to him – he did not want any, but he did have some lunch. I made some sandwiches and he had a glass of water. We sat together at the table opposite each other. I tried to make

conversation. I was feeling pretty wretched, so was he. He looked dis-
tracted and dejected.

Q. How would you describe him at this time?

A. Oh, I just thought he had a broken heart. He really was very, very —
he had shrunk into himself. He looked as though he had shrunk,
but I had no idea at that stage of what he might do later, absolutely
no idea at all.

Q. Did you talk much at lunch?

A. No, no. He could not put two sentences together. He could not talk
at all.

Q. You said, I think, you were feeling unwell that day?

A. That is right.

Q. What did you do?

A. I went to go and have a lie down after lunch, which is something I
quite often did, just to cope with my arthritis. I said to him, 'What
are you going to do?' He said, 'I will probably go for my walk.'

Q. What time do you think you went upstairs, so far as you can
remember?

A. It would be about half past 1, quarter to 2 perhaps.

Q. Where was he at that time?

A. He went into his study. Then shortly after I had laid down he came
to ask me if I was okay. I said: 'Yes, I will be fine.' And then he
went to change into his jeans. He would be around the house in a
tracksuit or tracksuit bottoms during the day. So he went to change
and put on his shoes. Then I assumed he had left the house.

Q. Because he was going for a walk?

A. That is right. He had intended to go for this regular walk of his. He
had a bad back, so that was the strategy for that.

Q. And did he, in fact, go straight off for his walk?

A. Well, the phone rang a little bit later on and I assumed he had
left . . . and I was aware of David talking quietly on a phone.

Q. Where was he at this time?

A. In his study.

Q. Do you know what time this was?

A. Getting on for 3, I would think.

Q. And did Dr Kelly go out for his walk?

A. He had gone by 3.20.

Q. So between 3 and 3.20 he had gone for a walk?

A. That is right, yes.

When he left the house, David Kelly met an elderly neighbour walking her dog. The neighbour was subsequently questioned.

Q. What did you say to him?

A. He said, 'Hello, Ruth,' and I said, 'Oh, hello, David, how are things?' He said, 'Not too bad.' We stood there for a few minutes, then Buster, my dog, was pulling on the lead, he wanted to get going. I said: 'I will have to go, David . . .' He said, 'See you again then, Ruth,' and that was it, we parted.

Q. How did he seem to you?

A. Just his normal self, no different to any other time when I have met him.

She was the last person to speak to David Kelly. He did not return from his walk. His wife was soon alarmed and their daughters arrived to search for him. Janice Kelly stated:

A. We had delayed calling the police because we thought we might make matters worse if David had returned when we started to search. I felt he was already in a difficult enough situation. So we put off calling the police until about 20 to 12 at night.

Q. The police are called. Do they turn up?

A. Three of them come with a missing persons form to fill in. I explained the situation that David had been in and it seemed immediately to go up to Chief Constable level . . . and the search begins. The Thames Valley helicopter had gone off duty by that time so they had to wait for the Benson helicopter to come across.

Q. That is RAF Benson, is it? So the helicopter was involved in searching?

A. And tracker dogs, too, I believe.

Q. Could you hear the helicopter?

A. Yes, it came and the police switched on their blue light on their vehicles so it could pinpoint the position of our house, the starting point for David's walk.

Q. Did you speak to the police at all during that night?

A. Yes, all night, all night. Then a vehicle arrived with a large communication mast on it and parked in the road and then during the early hours another mast, a 45-foot mast was put up in our garden.

Q. For police communications?

A. Yes, indeed. And a dog was put through our house. At 20 to 5 the following morning I was sitting on the lawn in my dressing gown while the dog went through the house.

I have read the reports of many such hideous nights of worry for the relatives of someone missing whose death by suicide is suspected. They try to cherish some sort of hope when, I believe, unacknowledged in their conscious minds, they know the truth. Mrs Kelly's misery and sickness in the hours leading up to her husband's death, before he had even left the house, perhaps indicate some intuition of what was to come, and her horror at it.

About forty officers were involved in the search, some with specialist knowledge of the area. Also, there were volunteers from a local association of dog owners whose animals have been trained for search and rescue. At about nine fifteen the next morning, one of these dogs located the body of David Kelly. The dog's owner found him in the woods where he often walked, and her description on finding him is important.

A. He was at the base of the tree with almost [sic] his head and his shoulders just slumped back against the tree.

Q. And what about his legs and arms? Where were they?

A. His legs were straight in front of him. His right arm was to the side of him. His left arm had a lot of blood on it and was bent back in a funny position.

Q. Did you see any blood anywhere else?

A. Just on the left arm and the left side.

Q. Could you tell whether or not this was the person you had been asked to look for?

A. Yes, the person matched the description that we had been given.

It was apparent to her that David Kelly was dead and there was nothing she could do to help him. She retraced her steps away from the body and her co-volunteer tried to call the police search team. He did not want to get close enough to the body to contaminate any evidence at the scene and so looked from a distance.

They were told to return to their car, which was about ten minutes away, and meet the police there. In fact, about two or three minutes later, they bumped into two detectives who had also begun to suspect that the body might be in this area. Of course, the detectives accompanied the volunteers straight back to David Kelly. The two search and rescue dog owners were not asked this question directly at the Hutton Inquiry, but my reading is that the body can only have been alone for a few minutes before they returned. Detective Constable Coe, however, describes the scene slightly differently.

Q. And how was the body positioned?

A. It was laying on its back – the body was laying on its back by a large tree, the head towards the trunk of the tree.

Q. Did you notice anything about the body?

A. I did.

Q. What did you notice?

A. I noticed that there was blood round the left wrist. I saw a knife, like a pruning knife, and a watch.

Q. And was the body lying on its front or on its back?

A. On its back.

Q. Where was the watch?

A. If I remember rightly, just on top of the knife.

Q. And where was the knife?

A. Near to the left wrist, left side of the body . . .

Q. Did you notice if there were any stains on the clothes?

A. I saw blood around the left wrist area.

Q. Anywhere else? How close an examination did you yourself make?

A. Just standing upright, I did not go over to the body . . . I observed the scene.

Q. How far away from the body did you actually go?

A. 7 or 8 feet.

Q. How long did you spend at the scene?

A. Until other officers came to tape off the area. I would think somewhere in the region of about 25 or 30 minutes.

I cannot personally explain the conflicting descriptions of the body's position. They have certainly fuelled many a conspiracy theory. The assumption of some commentators is that David Kelly was slumped against the tree when found as described and that someone then moved him in those few minutes, exact number unknown, when the volunteers were away meeting the police.

The evidence against this theory is conclusive to me. Until they encountered the detectives, the two volunteers did not see or hear anyone else in the woods, nor did the dog pick up any other human scent. I have closely examined all photos of the scene, both before and after the removal of the body, and there is no evidence at all of dragging. Pulling a heavy body across such soft, leaf-covered ground, or moving it at all, would certainly leave marks. Plus, the blood I see on the ground indicates that David Kelly was lying in the place and position in which he died.

By the time an ambulance arrived, there were many police around and a path from the road to the body had been staked out. The paramedics placed four electrodes on David Kelly's chest to verify that life was extinct. The monitor showed only a flat line. At the Hutton Inquiry, the first paramedic made the following point and it was later reiterated by the second.

Q. And is there anything else that you know of about the circumstances of Dr Kelly's death that you can assist his Lordship with?

A. Only that the amount of blood that was around the scene seemed relatively minimal and there was a small patch on his right knee, but no obvious arterial bleeding. There was no spraying of blood or huge blood loss or any obvious loss on the clothing.

Q. One of the police officers said there appeared to be some blood on the ground. Did you see that?

A. I could see some on — there were some stinging nettles to the left of the body. As to on the ground, I do not remember seeing a sort of huge puddle or anything like that. There was dried blood on the left wrist . . . but no obvious sign of a wound or anything, it was just dried blood.

Q. You did not see the wound?

A. I did not see the wound, no . . . The hand – from what I remember, his arm – left arm was outstretched to the left of the body . . . Palm up or slightly on the side [indicates] . . . dried blood from the edge of the jacket down towards the hand but no gaping wound or anything obvious that I could see from the position I was in.

Q. Were you examining the wrist for –

A. No, I was not. No.

Q. And were you examining the ground for blood or blood loss?

A. No.

These words added further fuel to the conspiracy theories, despite the fact that neither paramedic specifically examined David Kelly's arm or the ground around him. The most widespread theory goes like this. There was not enough blood at the scene to explain this death because he had been murdered in a different spot and placed there. The murder was made to look like suicide.

There is no implication here that a man was picked at random by a stranger while out walking. The implication is that David Kelly exposed government lies – lies which the government had spun to justify the UK's invasion of Iraq – and that consequently his murder was ordered.

It is a fact that no weapons of mass destruction were ever found in Iraq, let alone weapons that could be unleashed in forty-five minutes. The Chilcot Inquiry into the war, which was not published until 2016, used temperate language to damn the famous September dossier:

[The intelligence services reports] . . . contain careful language intended to ensure that no more weight is put on the evidence than it can bear. Organising the evidence in order to present an argument in the language of Ministerial

statements produces a quite different type of document . . .
Intelligence and assessments were used to prepare material
to be used to support Government statements in a way
which conveyed certainty without acknowledging the limitations of the intelligence.

Lord Chilcot went on to highlight the way the September
dossier had influenced public opinion.

The widespread perception that the September 2002 dossier overstated the firmness of the evidence about Iraq's
capabilities and intentions in order to influence opinion
and 'make the case' for action to disarm Iraq has produced a damaging legacy, including undermining trust and
confidence in Government statements, particularly those
which rely on intelligence which cannot be independently
verified.

David Kelly certainly played a role in that widespread perception with its damaging legacy and no doubt he greatly
annoyed the government. But does that give credibility to
claims that he was murdered? Let's go back to the woods
now where, at around 10 a.m. on 18 July, the paramedics cer-
tified his death.

Assistant Chief Constable Page was put in charge of the
investigation that day. He said:

We determined from the outset . . . that we would apply the
highest standards of investigation to this particular set of
circumstances as was possible. I would not say I launched
a murder investigation but the investigation was of that
standard.

After establishing a common approach path, the officers created a ten-metre-diameter circle around the body and within that circle they conducted a fingertip search. No one touched the body: the police wanted the forensic pathologist and forensic biologists to see everything exactly as found. Assistant Chief Constable Page said:

> . . . when I first saw Dr Kelly I was very aware of the serious nature of the search and I was looking for signs of perhaps a struggle; but all the vegetation that was surrounding Dr Kelly's body was standing upright and there were no signs of any form of struggle at all.

When the forensic pathologist, Dr Nicholas Hunt, arrived at 1235, he initially only confirmed death. He did not take David Kelly's temperature or examine him further but withdrew to await the biologist and his assistant, who were going to examine the scene. He was finally logged into the search area again at just after 1400, by which time there was a tent in position over the body. One of the many challenges to this case has come from people who think it suspicious that Dr Hunt did not take the body temperature on arrival, body temperature being considered essential information when estimating time of death. But his reasons for doing so were the right reasons: he would have had to remove clothing and this would have been impossible without causing any disturbance while the scene was still under close examination.

David Kelly was first examined forensically for fibres, fingerprints and other trace evidence and then Dr Hunt removed the clothes.

A. [He] . . . was wearing a green Barbour type wax jacket and the zip and the buttons at the front had been undone. Within the bellows pocket on the lower part of the jacket there was a mobile telephone and a pair of bi-focal spectacles. There was a key fob and, perhaps more significantly, a total of three blister packs of a drug called coproxamol. Each of those packs would originally have contained 10 tablets, a total of 30 potentially available.
Q. And how many tablets were left in those packs?
A. There was one left.

Now that the clothing could be properly examined, Dr Hunt noted extensive bloodstaining: over the front of the shirt, over the Barbour jacket, including the left sleeve, on the trousers over the right knee. David Kelly's arms were stained, especially the left. So was the back of the left elbow and the palm and fingers of the right hand. The blood-stained knife was by his left hand; so was his bloodstained wristwatch.

Q. Was there any other blood-staining that you noticed in the area?
A. There was an area of blood-staining to his left side running across the undergrowth and the soil, and I estimated it was over an area of 2 to 3 feet in maximum length.
Q. Did you carry out any particular tests of the scene?
A. Yes. In addition to the trace evidence gathering I also, having completed that, carried out a rectal temperature assessment.
Q. What time did you carry that out?
A. That reading was made at 19.15 hours.

Despite widespread criticism, all the evidence is that David Kelly's death was treated with the protocols, caution and forensic care of a potential homicide. The length and detailed nature of the scene examination, the extensive sampling for later scientific analysis, it was all designed to establish whether anyone had been near the deceased at the time of his death, and particularly whether there had been a struggle. The fact that body temperature was not taken until 1915 is also entirely in order: it reflects the meticulous nature of the scene and body examination until that time.

The body was then removed in a sealed body bag containing inner plastic sheeting to prevent contamination or unauthorized handling. The post-mortem began before witnesses at 2120 hours in the fully equipped mortuary at the John Radcliffe Hospital in Oxford. There was a very high degree of dissection, which is performed only in suspicious cases, so that all injuries, even those not visible on the skin surface, can be identified. As well as the obvious injuries to the wrist, which included a severed artery, there were some small grazes on the left side of the head, small areas of bruising on the left shin and below the right knee, on the lower part of the left side of the chest and in the right lower back.

These minimal injuries are certainly insufficient to suggest that David Kelly, an active, middle-aged man, had been physically restrained. Not before, during or after death. Nor does he seem to have been incapacitated by a third party: despite careful searching, no injection sites were discovered and there were no marks on the skin that might have come from an electrical stun device such as a Taser.

However, there was one surprising discovery at the post-mortem. David Kelly had suffered from advanced disease of the coronary arteries. In fact, there was evidence that the blockages in his coronary arteries had caused small heart attacks in the past. He had not visited a doctor and had probably assumed he was suffering from indigestion.

The coronary arteries feed the heart, and the right coronary artery was almost completely blocked in one place. You might think that must certainly kill you, since blood and therefore oxygen would not have been able to reach the heart to keep it beating. And indeed it might, unless the blockage has developed slowly, over some years. In that case, collateral blood vessels have time to develop around the blockage and blood is supplied to the heart muscle through them. Think how congested local roads become after a motorway closure. And how much smaller these roads are, how indirect the route can be to one's destination and how much less predictable and reliable travel now becomes – even though it is still possible.

Another major coronary artery, the left anterior descending, was 60 to 70 per cent blocked and, indeed, blockages in this artery are one of Western society's biggest killers. The last of the heart's three major blood suppliers, the circumflex artery, had similarly narrowed. The fact is that David Kelly apparently had no knowledge of his heart disease but it was so advanced that he could have died of natural causes at any time.

Did this disease play a role in his death?

As bleeding from his wrist injury continued and his circulating blood volume fell, adrenaline would have kicked in. This maintains blood pressure by constricting non-essential blood vessels all around the body – but it dilates the arteries to the heart. As it does so, the heart rate increases. The heart is working harder and so needs more oxygen from an increased blood flow – but with such diseased coronary arteries, the heart would have received little of the necessary

259

increase. One constituent of the co-proxamol painkillers he took, probably to limit the pain from cutting his wrist, might also have had an effect on his heart. This constituent can cause abnormalities of rhythm, especially where blood pressure is low. So it is very possible that death was hastened, but not caused, by David Kelly's cardiovascular disease.

The fact that he had apparently not been complaining of any significant cardiac problems, despite his serious, underlying medical condition, is not at all unusual. He may well have had no symptoms. Or he may simply have been stoical in the face of symptoms, explaining them away. Or he may have had a complete lack of interest in his own wellbeing due to stress or depression.

Dr Hunt gave as cause of death:

1a. Haemorrhage
1b. Incised wounds to the left wrist
  2. Co-proxamol ingestion and coronary artery atherosclerosis.

I totally agree with him. But alternative theories about the death of David Kelly from a wide body of people, including a few medics, have never gone away.

Here are my responses to some of the many criticisms and challenges to Dr Hunt's conclusion.

- David Kelly was right-handed, according to his family. Right-handed people preferentially inflict injuries to their left wrists. And to do so they remove clothing or other artefacts that might get in the way. David Kelly's wristwatch lay on the ground beside him. Few murderers would have been so thoughtful or so neat.

- It is certainly possible to die from the severing of the ulnar artery in the wrist, as from the severing of any artery. The doctors who have shed doubt on this are doctors of the living, not the dead, and perhaps they have treated ulnar arteries severed by accident rather than by suicide. After an isolated, accidental wrist injury, there is usually someone at hand who will try to stem the blood flow; many lay people have the knowledge or the instinct to make a tourniquet. Someone in the act of suicide does nothing to stem the flow. In fact, exactly the opposite. The suicidal are actually likely to manipulate the wound to maximize blood loss and might also take active measures, like flexing the wrist, to prevent any clotting.
- The knife found with the deceased was entirely capable of causing the incised injuries to the wrist. People demand: why are there no fingerprints on it? Because there seldom are. We use knives with the middle of our fingers, not the pads, which leave prints. However, if I killed someone and wanted to fake their suicide, I would personally still try to make sure their prints were left on the knife.
- Dr Hunt has been accused of not applying certain factors when calculating time of death. This is true, he did not. But the estimation of the time of any death is already so variable and flawed that I think this is totally irrelevant. Time, body temperature and ambient temperature and a plethora of other factors may, or may not, play a part.

The accusation is that Dr Hunt failed to allow for David Kelly's layers of clothing. But let's remember that a full night followed by the next day, with its July heat, had come and gone before Dr Kelly's temperature was taken – and by that time his body was covered by a tent in which people were working. Also, loss of blood may well lead to loss of heat. A plethora of factors indeed.

And even when all the factors are considered, every 't' crossed and every 'i' dotted, then the very best estimate that a pathologist can reach covers a time span of over five hours. So much for 'the' time of death.

The reason I don't think Dr Hunt's slight miscalculation matters is this. Most forensic pathologists use a nomogram designed by Claus Henssge to calculate time of death. I am going to make an immodest claim for myself now. While examining Dr Hunt's results in the David Kelly case, I spotted a printing error of Henssge's nomogram in the UK standard textbook of forensic pathology, the source of the nomogram we all rely on to estimate time of death.

Henssge's nomogram looks a bit like a mysterious astrological chart, with its complexity of concentric rings, lines and numbers. I realized that the printers of the textbook had tweaked the nomogram to fit neatly on to the page. The change was subtle but, for practical purposes, this change completely distorted the chart, making our results from it useless. And I mean everyone's results in every case where that version of the nomogram had been used. As we nearly all used this same textbook, the cases affected by this discovery were numerous.

I wrote to the Home Office, and much commotion ensued. All cases where time of death was a significant factor in the determination of guilt or innocence had to be reviewed. And we forensic pathologists all now have to consult a different edition of the nomogram. The Home Office's letter to my colleagues began: 'Someone has noticed that . . .' I'm trying to keep my ego under control. But I wish it had said: 'Dr Richard Shepherd has noticed that . . .' because I do consider spotting this error perhaps my greatest (my only? I hope not) contribution to forensic pathology.

Anyway, Dr Hunt was almost certainly using the distorted nomogram, like nearly all of us. And he may also have been working from a photocopy of the book – which we soon realized causes further marginal distortion. In fact, in all later editions of the textbook there is a note, in red, next to the nomogram, advising that copies are not to be used for calculations.

So accusations that Dr Hunt's estimation of the time of death was wrong may be correct – but who could possibly know? In the circumstances, he gave the best estimate that he could, and he cannot be blamed for either the variability in the way the human body cools after death, or indeed for the printing error of the chart. Neither of which points to a conspiracy.

- Some critics have claimed that David Kelly could not have consumed so many co-proxamol tablets to relieve his pain by using the small amount of water in his nearby bottle of Evian. But, in my opinion, it is easily possible to ingest twenty-nine tablets using only 300 ml of water.
- I can't explain why the first people to find the body said he was slumped against the tree when in the subsequent photos of the scene he clearly wasn't. But neither can I find any forensic evidence that he

was moved, especially since the body, once discovered, was unattended only for a few minutes. Divergence of apparently reliable eyewitness evidence seems to have been a feature of every trial I have been involved in. Without it, how would barristers earn their money? It has always seemed to me that it is the concurrence of such evidence in TV crime dramas that makes them so unbelievable.

- I don't agree with some critics who say that blood from the scene should have been quantified by recovering the vegetation, soil and leaf litter on the ground. I have never done this and never known it to be done. It seems impractical and unscientific to me and the blood in vegetation certainly isn't measurable with any precision. This criticism must be prompted by the concern of the ambulance personnel that there was not enough evidence of blood. But they admitted that they quite correctly did not fully examine the body or the scene. Nor would it have been possible for them to know how much blood had seeped into the soil. Dr Hunt, on the other hand, did carry out this examination and he did see a lot of blood at the scene and on the clothing.

- I can deduce from the pictures of the scene that David Kelly vomited twice when he started bleeding: the areas of vomiting lie to the side of his left shoulder and head. The bloodstaining of the right knee of his jeans would be consistent with him turning to his left side and kneeling in order to vomit at these sites. I don't believe that the number of tablets he took could or should have been established by examining the vomit, as some people have suggested. Full toxicology analysis was carried out on David Kelly's blood to determine the number of painkillers he took.

- There is a suggestion that, following an old injury, Dr Kelly would not have had the strength in his right arm to sever an artery. I could find nothing in his medical records to suggest that the injury had not healed, perhaps with a little restricted movement. After death, it is of course impossible to determine muscle strength, but certainly no evidence of muscle wastage was found in the right arm.

- Dr Kelly's weight at post-mortem was recorded at 59 kg, when, shortly before his death, his weight was recorded at 79 kg. Most of this difference can be easily explained. First, because in life he was almost certainly weighed with his clothes on. Second, because blood weighs over 1 kg a litre and so significant blood loss would result in a much lower body weight. The third reason is prosaic. Mortuary scales are notoriously inaccurate.

- I should also remind you that David Kelly's glasses were found in his pocket, along with the empty blister packs of painkillers. I think it unlikely that an individual who had been attacked would take off his glasses and place them in his pocket before he was killed, and I have never known an assailant do that either.

I think I am asked about the death of Dr David Kelly more often than about any other death and, whenever I say that it was caused, I do not doubt, by his suicide, the temperature in the room is guaranteed to drop a few degrees. His name has become synonymous not, sadly, with his distinguished career, but with allegations of a government cover-up.

One of two governments is generally considered by theorists to be responsible for his death. First, he was accused of being a spy for Russia and there is a theory that the Russian government chose to dispose of him. I can only say that the scenario of a faked suicide in the woods is a long way from Alexander Litvinenko's death (poisoned by Polonium 210 in 2006), or Sergei Skripal's near death (poisoned by Novichok in 2018).

More often, though, the British government is blamed. Personally, I cannot see what the government might have gained from such a murder. Dr Kelly had already been 'thrown to the wolves', as one of those wolves had suggested to him during his appearance before the Foreign Affairs Committee. Why blame the government for his murder when they could and perhaps should be blamed instead for disgracing someone who had served them well for many years, and discarding him in a manner which led to his suicide? Isn't that bad enough?

I had all these thoughts about the context of David Kelly's death when giving my case review. Of course, it is hard not to form a personal opinion on the reported background events. But I have to ignore that and draw my medico-legal conclusions from the forensic facts only. And the forensic facts point one way. To suicide.

I doubt my analysis here will do much to stem the conspiracy theories. They have such an enduring power. Too enduring for the suffering Kelly family, who, according to some newspaper reports, have recently had David Kelly's body exhumed, cremated and reburied elsewhere after there was evidence of tampering at the grave.

We can learn little about conspiracies and a lot about suicide from David Kelly's death. His family's description of his behaviour in his final weeks of life is both moving and recognizable to anyone who has weathered a suicide in their circle. Here we find a man who saw no other escape from an escalating situation – remember, he had on the morning of his death received notice of four parliamentary questions designed, with what seem to me and must have seemed to him, vindictive intent, to ensure he was publicly reprimanded. After that, perhaps it also appeared to Dr Kelly that his former life could never be recovered.

An important witness at the Hutton Inquiry into David Kelly's death was Professor Hawton, psychiatrist and director of Oxford University's Centre for Suicide Research. He was asked how it was that the neighbour who had passed David Kelly as he walked to the woods to kill himself had given evidence that he was behaving normally.

A. Well, I think it is consistent with the notion that he had made a decision before that to end his life . . . certainly it is not an unusual experience . . . for people who come into contact with [someone who is near to ending their life] to say that they seemed actually better than they had been . . . before . . . And I think it is this – it is having, in a sense, decided on how to deal with the problem, that leads to a sort of sense of peace and calm . . .

Q. And what styles of thinking are most associated with suicide?

A. Well, the one for which there is most evidence is the tendency to feel hopeless when faced with a difficult circumstance . . . a sense of feeling trapped, being unable to escape from an unbearable situation. Isolation may be another factor, either actual isolation in the sense of not having people around or relative isolation where a person is unable to communicate with those around them because of their particular personality style.

Q. We have heard that [Dr Kelly] was a weapons inspector, it must have put him in all sorts of difficult situations. Was that similar to the situation that he found himself in towards the end of his life?

A. No, I think there was an important difference. One has heard about the situations he faced, for example, in Iraq, while cross-examining people, which sounded to me quite terrifying situations. I gather he could cope with those extremely well. I think the importance about the problems he was facing shortly before his death was that these really challenged his identity of himself, his self-esteem, his self-worth, his image of himself as a valued and loyal employee and as a significant scientist . . . as far as one can deduce, the major factor [in his suicide] was the severe loss of self-esteem, resulting from his feeling that people had lost trust in him and from his dismay at being exposed to the media.

Q. And why have you singled that out as a major factor?

A. Well . . . I think being such a private man, I think this was anathema to him to be exposed, you know, publicly in this way. In a sense, I think he would have seen it as being publicly disgraced . . . I think another very relevant factor . . . was his private nature, his dislike of sharing personal problems and feelings with other people; and according to several accounts, he had become increasingly withdrawn into himself during the period shortly before his death which meant that I think he became even less accessible or less able to discuss his problems with other people.

Q. What other factors do you think were relevant?

A. I think that, carrying on that theme, I think he must have begun . . . to think that, first of all, the prospects for continuing in his previous work role were diminishing very markedly and, indeed, my conjecture is that he had begun to fear he would lose his job altogether.

Q. What effect is that likely to have had on him?

*A. I think that would have filled him with a profound sense of hope-
lessness; and that, in a sense, his life's work had been not wasted but
that it had been totally undermined.*

There is no forensic evidence that points to murder rather
than suicide in David Kelly's case. But the most compelling
evidence that he ended his own life is here, in Professor
Hawton's testimony and that of the Kelly family. His was a
tragic case of classic, middle-aged male suicide. The involvement of the government and the national importance of his
actions in the last few months of his life does nothing to
change the fact that his trajectory towards death was characteristic of a crisis many people encounter, particularly in
midlife.

The sixth age shifts
Into the lean and slipper'd pantaloon;
With spectacles on nose and pouch on side;
His youthful hose, well sav'd, a world too wide
For his shrunk shank; and his big manly voice,
Turning again toward childish treble, pipes
And whistles in his sound:

15

Alfred Hoop was sixty-six years old. He was short and decidedly stocky. His hair was grey, but he had little of it left. His face, although rather a mess at the moment, was clean-shaven. His fingers were nicotine-stained. He was missing a number of teeth, which, despite some replacements, must have been obvious whenever he smiled. He was tattooed on the right upper arm and both forearms. In men of his age, this sometimes points to a maritime connection and I thought perhaps he was an old sailor. A note from a police officer confirmed that he had been a docker in his youth and, when the last of the docks had closed in London, he worked on building sites. He had retired a year ago but sometimes returned to help out for cash in hand.

His body told the story of an eventful and occasionally violent life. One eye had the strange milkiness of partial opacity. There was a host of surgical scars on his abdomen, chest and neck. How easy it would have been to conclude that he had been the victim of one terrible accident. Except that the scars were of various ages.

When his medical notes arrived, they revealed that his forties had been his most difficult decade. At forty-three, he had been involved in a road traffic accident which left him with quite serious chest injuries. Alfred bounced back but, soon after that, he was stopped while driving erratically by the police. They must have thought they had apprehended a drunk, but Alfred was sober. The police discovered he could not see at all with one eye. Investigation revealed that an accident in his twenties – not detailed – had left him with corneal scarring and that over the years he had gradually lost his sight. Sight is a strange thing: the brain adjusts for its deficiencies and it is possible to lose a lot of vision without really knowing it. Or perhaps Alfred had known but not admitted it to himself. The eye was described as unseeing and 'cosmetically unattractive'.

At forty-seven, he had been stabbed in the back. His notes gave no further details.

Over the years, Alfred, typically of those who do hard, physical work, had sustained minor injuries. In his case, there were many, from a fractured elbow caused by a fall to an infected wound caused by treading on a nail. He had repeatedly requested sick notes from the doctor and had quite often needed antibiotics for infections, usually resulting from small, work-related misfortunes.

I felt it was fair to assume that Alfred's work had been arduous and that he had been a fighting man. Apart from all the wounds and scars, he had the physique of someone who had, earlier in life, been very strong and fit. Now, however, he was carrying a good few extra kilos. Even though he was just sixty-six, he looked like an old man.

When does middle age stop and old age begin? By dividing middle age into early and late, I had hoped to persuade the reader that late middle age might these days include at least the early, even the mid-sixties. But I'm no longer in my mid-sixties and by now I should have recognized a fact no one of my generation, and Alfred's, likes at all. We call ourselves baby boomers to avoid saying it. I am old. We are old. And from here it's downhill all the way.

I daresay that Alfred Hoop did not regard himself as old,

and it is entirely possible that when those of us who are over sixty look in the mirror we see our younger selves. The most obvious indicator of age is weight gain and, like Alfred, I am expanding. I hope no one would describe me as fat but, in the few years since semi-retirement, I have piled on kilos and my BMI is now 27, an unhealthy two notches over the upper limit of normal. So I am officially 'overweight' for the first time in my life. I am aware of the risks of being overweight, greatly increased now by Covid-19, but I have, as yet, devoted no large amount of time to tackling this.

I notice that other people in this age group study their health and discuss it at every opportunity. Baby boomers have funded a new self-care industry. We spend a not insignificant propor- tion of life trying to prolong it and prolong its quality, and we can only hope that time spent on maintenance does not exceed the time this earns us. I'm talking about the dentistry, the hygienist, the flossing, the gum stimulators, the expensive toothbrushes, the chiropodist, the orthotic shoe inserts, the hair treatments, the Botox, the plastic surgery, the health screening, the ergonomic chairs, the special reading lamps, the osteopath, the chiropractor, the optician, the prescription sun- glasses, glasses, contact lenses, the support socks, the knee braces, the yoga classes, the magnetic therapy bracelets . . . and all this for people who probably feel quite well. Many in this age group, and I do not mean just the wealthy, are leaving the work- force now and they are spending much of their retirement and their pensions keeping decline at bay.

Despite all this attention to self, we are failing miserably in the fundamentals: specifically, only a minority of us maintain a healthy weight. In the sixty-six to seventy-four age group, three quarters of us are obese or overweight. Younger baby boomers are not faring much better, but those of us born after the war but before the mid-1950s are the fattest and we are most likely to be admitted to hospital for causes directly or indirectly related to obesity. We are financed in this, of course, by younger taxpayers.

There is much inequality in obesity, whatever your age. Certain ethnicities, low income and leaving school early are all associated with higher weight. Men are more likely to be overweight than women, but women are more likely to be obese than men. And a significantly higher proportion of women have large waists. This is important because waist circumference is considered a good indicator of the risk of diabetes, cardiovascular disease and many other health problems. A desirable waist size is under 80 cm for women and under 94 cm for men. If that sounds absurd for the very tall, then a waistline which is half your height is healthy enough. Among baby boomers, 85 per cent of women and 74 per cent of men out-bulge any healthy circumference and, once again, I am sorry to find myself, although only recently, with the majority.

We are a cohort of Falstaffs, but we baby boomers were almost certainly slim as children – childhood obesity rates in that era were minuscule and we need only look at old family photographs to confirm how skinny we were. We were probably slim well into adulthood, too. My own professional files start in 1987, and the bodies photographed then show a population so slender that I can hardly believe we are the same nation – and this is irrespective of the deceased's age or cause of death. When baby boomers were young they were cared for by adults who were certainly an inch or two shorter than adults today but very much lighter: fathers then weighed on average just 65 kg (10.2 stone) and mothers 55 kg (8.7 stone). Only a tiny percentage were obese.

The whole nation has gained weight, and we know why.

The picture is sometimes complex but, put simply, the cause must be our sedentary lifestyles and our access to cheap, pre-prepared food, much of which hides a very high fat and sugar content because it is designed to please us and bring us back for more. But we are not all equally fat. The graphs show a steady increase in weight as we get older. Is this inevitable? And is my cohort the fattest simply because ours is the last age group before senility and shrinkage set in?

There are some physical and metabolic reasons why weight gain is easier as we age, but the basic equation between calories in and calories burnt remains the same. Getting older seldom means we eat less, but we usually do less. How many sixty-five-year-olds do you know who bound upstairs? Exercise, if we take it at all, is probably compartmentalized into the daily walk instead of an intrinsic component of everyday life, and Covid-19's lockdowns have exacerbated this habit. We burn fewer calories because we are simply more sedentary, perhaps because exercise hurts in places it never used to, and we do not adjust our food intake. The fundamental explanation for weight gain in my age group must be this: a failure or a refusal to recognize that we have changed.

This lack of recognition of the limitations ageing brings is hazardous. Perhaps people put on weight and ignore it. Or they are so alarmed by weight gain that they return to a form of exercise they enjoyed twenty, or even just ten years ago. Only to find, through some painful injury, that they cannot recapture their ten-years-ago self. Loss of a younger self is hard enough, but the results of failing to recognize this loss are harsher. Alfred Hoop had died in a fight at sixty-six, but his body spoke of many fights long ago: had he perhaps fallen victim to an old man's delusion of youthfulness?

His liver was in very good condition, so it was not safe to

assume that his fighting past had been due to drinking. Perhaps he had been a man of very quick temper, or perhaps he had given up alcohol long ago, before his input exceeded his liver's ability to repair itself.

He did not smell of alcohol, but the police in the post-mortem room were sure that the toxicologist would find some significant alcohol intake. They were holding three big lads in custody and, for them, Alfred's demise felt like another of the boozy punch-ups they attend so often. I sensed a certain malaise. Another drunk, another fight, another death.

Until a detective arrived with the details and some witness statements. When he told the story, the mood of the assembled officers changed entirely, from a certain bored indifference to something much softer and much sadder.

Alfred had a handicapped son in his thirties who had a mental age of eight. Evidently, it was easy to tell from the son's demeanour that he was different. Some people respond to this with empathy and others, unfortunately, see it as a weakness to be exploited, either by ridicule or aggression.

Alfred and his wife had taken very good care of their son: in court Alfred was spoken of as a gentle, loving and kind father. On the day of his death he had taken his son to a music concert for a treat. As they queued outside the well-known venue, three large lads approached his son and demanded a cigarette from him. He did not have a cigarette and this greatly angered the lads, who began to jeer at him. Then they started to push him, unreasonably and aggressively demanding an apology for his failure to supply them with nicotine.

The son blabbered constant, terrified apologies, but by now the bullies were punching him. Alfred immediately squared up to them – the old fighter, who must fight again.

Years ago, he would probably have been quick enough and strong enough to take on three lads. But not now. No one can blame him for defending his son, but it is no surprise, given the youth and aggression of the perpetrators, that he was rapidly knocked to the ground. Eyewitnesses said that the lads then stamped on his head and chest.

The police arrived before the ambulance. Alfred's face was covered in blood and they found no pulse. They attempted resuscitation without success, then rolled him on to his side, and one of the officers scooped out some debris and fluid from his mouth. They started resuscitation again and this time heard gurgling, rasping noises from within Alfred's chest – a positive sign. And, indeed, his chest started rising and falling again. Until, a few minutes later, it stopped.

'There appeared to be a blockage and we were unable to inflate his chest now,' said their report, significantly. They rolled him again, cleared his mouth again, and kept trying CPR. The ambulance soon arrived.

The paramedics also gave statements. One said: 'I was informed by the police officer that he was struggling to get an airway and there had been debris in the mouth, which he had cleared . . . I would say that, compared to the pub punchups I have attended, this elderly man's injuries were ten-fold worse, the severity of the bruising was horrific, and I can remember feeling quite shocked.'

Inside the ambulance, the paramedics used all means at their disposal to get a pulse, and at first they seemed to succeed: they then rushed to the hospital, a paramedic and a police officer carrying out CPR all the way. However, although there was a pulse, Alfred was not breathing on his own. Hospital staff were standing by to receive the patient and, after doing all they could, transferred him to the nearest hospital which had a bed available in the intensive care unit.

The ICU doctor writes:

It was immediately apparent that Mr Hoop had sustained a severe injury to his brain. He was comatose and unresponsive to pain ... we concluded that the injury was due to anoxia (shortage of oxygen) to the brain caused either by cardiac arrest or head injury. I made the family aware of how serious the situation was and advised them of three possibilities. First, we believed that Mr Hoop had underlying heart disease and therefore it was likely that the assault had caused a heart attack. Second, that bleeding in his body had stopped oxygen reaching his heart, resulting in a cardiac arrest. The third was that his head injury had caused him to lose consciousness and that consequent breathing difficulties had caused a cardiac arrest.

Let the doctors of the living speculate. A doctor of the dead like me can open the body and solve mysteries. At least, I thought so.

Alfred's heart stopped and was restarted once more in ICU before the doctors told the family that further resuscitation was inadvisable. He died about twenty-four hours after the assault. And now that the police knew the whole story and had the three lads in custody, they were keen to press charges.

It did occur to me that we had all misjudged Alfred by his tough, docker's exterior. The police thought he had got into a drunken brawl – now this had patently been proved wrong, especially when the tox report showed that he had taken no drink at all. I had assumed, from his physique and his scars, that he was a pugnacious man whose quick temper tended to get him into trouble, but soon there was a mountain of witness statements all saying that Alfred had spent a long time pleading with his son's attackers before he finally returned their blows. And the ICU doctors suspected that, because Alfred was overweight and a smoker, he had some underlying heart disease that had precipitated death in the circumstances. But, when I examined Alfred's heart, I found it to be in very good condition: there was no sign of any previous heart attack, no enlargement to suggest the heart had been struggling, the valves were healthy and so was the pericardium. Not only that but, for a man of his age, the atheroma in his arteries was remarkably minimal – although, having lived in an industrialized part of east London and smoked twenty a day for many years, he did have emphysema (a long-term and worsening lung condition which is now classified as part of the catch-all Chronic Obstructive Pulmonary Disease). I myself had judged him externally to be an old man. Inside his body, senescence was far from advanced.

In other words, we all made many assumptions about Alfred based on his external appearance which internal examination did not support. A lesson I find I must constantly relearn.

But how had Alfred actually died? Some of the bruising on his face was due to punches, I was sure, but the rest was very likely stamping – you could see something close to a shoe print in the blood. This must surely have contributed to his death. There were no other head injuries. He had apparently fallen backwards, and this is very often fatal, but he showed no laceration. A mystery.

When I examined some of Alfred's organs under a microscope, I began to suspect a possible cause of death, and it had nothing to do with his head, although the hospital doctors had been certain of serious brain injury. Despite the lack of evidence for this, my next job was to ask a neuropathologist to examine his brain. She concluded that he had widespread brain damage from lack of oxygen but that he had definitely not sustained a traumatic head injury.

So now I was sure. Alfred's lungs had shown evidence of acute aspiration and aspiration pneumonia. This is an infection which can occur very rapidly if something supposed to be in our digestive system finds its way to our respiratory system.

Aspiration certainly fitted with the police officers' description of removing debris from Alfred's airway and how the airway seemed to become blocked again. I felt sure that the so-called debris was actually vomit. It is not unusual to vomit after receiving a blow. Vomit is an acidic irritant if it reaches our breathing apparatus: food or any foreign object can rapidly infect the lungs, but a healthy person swallows, coughs or gags to force the food out, or if they are lucky a first-aider helps them by using the Heimlich manoeuvre. Alfred was not lucky, and he could not swallow, cough or gag because he had been knocked unconscious. Vomit in the airways had obstructed them and had stopped oxygen getting to his brain and heart. As a result it had stopped beating – but it had been restarted. However, over the ensuing few hours, the residual trapped vomit had caused irritation of the airways and lungs and finally pneumonia. And this chain of events caused his death. I gave:

1a. **Cerebral anoxia**
1b. **Aspiration of gastric contents and pneumonia.**

His three young assailants now faced a murder charge and their defence team leapt gleefully on to my post-mortem report. They claimed that the hospital was at fault for not treating Alfred for bronchopneumonia and, even more strongly, they insisted that Alfred's emphysema had played a crucial role in its development. How, they argued, could the perpetrators have known of this weakness during a little horseplay?

Even the healthiest lungs can rapidly submit to infection, so this claim about the emphysema was medical nonsense. But suggesting nonsense has never in my experience been known to stop a defence barrister, as long as it can be made to sound feasible.

As is usual, I returned to the mortuary to re-examine Alfred's bruises in case any more had appeared a few days after death. And now I was asked to investigate another defence argument: it related to, very unusually, the victim's knees.

A witness had stated that Alfred had not been struck on to his knees but had sunk there, as if one knee had simply given way with arthritis. The witness had arthritis herself and had experienced a knee collapsing suddenly under her and she believed that Alfred had sunk to the ground during the fight in a similar manner. It would have been easy to dismiss this, except that I had already been surprised at the way Alfred had hit the ground without causing any laceration to the back of the head.

On my re-examination, I found that a few new bruises had appeared, but none of them made much difference to my report. I then opened his knees. Forensic pathologists are rarely asked to do this because there are few circumstances in which the knees are relevant to the facts of a case. Alfred's knees showed me that he did indeed have arthritis.

Arthritis is caused by wear and tear to the joints. Personally,

I suspected long ago, in my forties, that I was destined to experience this later in life in my weight-bearing joints. I had found two small lumps on the last joint of both index fingers. They remain there today and, following the medical habit of naming lumps and bumps, these are called Heberden's nodes. They are tiny bony growths, and I don't remember ever having pain associated with them, although for some people they are, apparently, painful. When these nodes first appeared, I regarded myself as an interesting case to observe. Now, I could establish whether or not it was just an old wives' tale that getting nodes in the fingers in middle age points to osteo-arthritis in the hips or knees developing later.

It wasn't an old wives' tale. I do indeed now have osteoarthritis in my knees. Arthritis, more than any other condition, cruelly extracts vengeance for the excesses and mistakes of our youth. The truth is that both I and Alfred Hoop, and perhaps most men of this age, sustained damage, for whatever reason, forty, fifty years or more before we were presented with the bill.

I may not have shone at school sports, but I enjoyed them. I daresay I took a few knocks. Once I'd left school, the greatest injury I risked was from drunken dancing as a student. But there is that excruciating stumble when running for a bus, that twist of the knee when kicking a ball with the kids . . . these are minor and rapidly forgotten incidents, but they can cause what seems like a temporary weakness in one place. Actually, that place remains an area of weakness, particularly if it is a knee. The knees are in daily use and often under strain. Repair is slow and greatly hampered by the constant stress the knee faces, and in the long term this is a battle which the knee cannot win. In my case, repair has been hampered on the one hand by many long hours of standing over a post-mortem table, and on the other by a lot of walking briskly up steep hills with dogs. For Alfred Hoop, who started a life of hard physical work in the days when there was little regard for health and safety, any number of small accidents and stresses must have occurred. He worked standing up, that is almost certain, and so his knees had no respite. And his later-life weight gain would have increased the burden on his knees still more.

The knee fights a losing battle, but still it fights. Once tissue is damaged, it sends out chemical signals that bring white cells rushing to repair it and other cells to clean up the debris. While the repair operation goes on, cartilage, the cushion between the bones in our knee joints, is nevertheless thinning at the point of weakness and damage. This shifts the load it carries, just a little, to the edge of the joint. The repair work shifts, too. At the edge of the joint, new cartilage is formed and this stimulates new bone growth where it is really not needed at all. And that is why osteoarthritis is characterized by bone thickening and small bony outcrops while, inside the joint, the cartilage is thinning. As usual, genes have a role to play here. Our work, play and overall weight have a direct effect on our cartilage – but maybe the ease with which it wears away is determined at least partly by genetic factors outside our control.

I can't, of course, see my own knee cartilage, but I expect it is distinctly worn in places. Cartilage is strange stuff. It is the colour of vodka and tonic: a sort of smoky grey, almost transparent. It looks as if it must be jelly, but try to cut it and it turns out to be very solid; in fact more like very strong plastic than jelly. It can be cut only with a decidedly sharp knife.

Healthy cartilage is 4 or 5 mm thick and very smooth, like a cricket pitch. The first sign of wear is a change in this appearance: no one is coming to mow the pitch. Gradually, the roughened surface thins in weak points. I've seen cartilage just 0.5 mm thick. In Alfred's right knee, his cartilage was as thin as 1.5 mm and in other places as thick as 5 mm. It was a bit like a moth-eaten rug, and there is nothing unusual about that in a sixty-six-year-old man. I suspect he wasn't the sort of person to complain a lot, but I bet his right knee hurt him sometimes, especially if he sat still for too long. I bet he was stiff when he got out of bed and that some mornings it took him a few minutes to persuade his knee that it wanted to walk.

How do I know that? Because one day, perhaps ten years ago, I knelt down to examine the scene of a crime and my knees hurt so much I had to stand up. It happened again. And then again. After that, there was no more kneeling. Some years later, I found that I was stiff when I got up from my chair or from bed, as if the knee joint was locked, although with a few minutes of activity it was fine. I knew that by now the cartilage must be getting more worn. The great smoothness required for knee efficiency was being lost: instead of sliding across ice, the two bones were hitting patches of earth where the ice had melted.

Of course, it has worsened. When I get up in the morning, I stand for a moment, waiting for my knees to give me permission to walk. Then I go downstairs, holding on to the bannister. Not gripping it. Not yet, anyway. My hand slides lightly. The same on the Underground escalators. I insinuate myself into the right-hand queue so that I will have a hand-rail. I know that, with so much less cartilage, my knees are beginning to become unstable and could collapse quite dramatically. They have not, yet, but it could happen. I don't believe I appear in any way doddery. I alone know that, inside my legs, are very old knees.

I am lucky that my arthritis is not painful yet. I would describe my knees as uncomfortable. Restricting. Annoying. But there is little pain. Further degeneration is likely. How can I keep it at bay? Developing the muscles around the knee gives it important support, and I shall continue to get plenty of exercise to prevent my knees from stiffening, even though I know that exercise is a contributing factor to arthritis. It's a balancing act, pitting the risks against the benefits. Perhaps that balancing act *is* old age.

What about the appearance of the arthritic bone, left behind and trying to function as cartilage disappears? Everyone assumes bone must be white because that's how skeletons are always portrayed, at Halloween or in anatomy class. Those skeletons have all been soaked in solvent and bleached. Bone is actually quite an unattractive shade of off-white, sometimes close to grey. Where the cartilage has worn so thin that it offers virtually no cushion, bone rubs on bone. This is a painful thought, reminding me of massive granite wheels grinding together in some ancient water mill.

After years of this, the bone becomes smooth and white with a yellowish sheen, like ivory. And in the places where cartilage was worn, Arthur's right knee had that ivory look, which is called eburnation.

His arthritis was bad in a few areas of one knee, but I had a horrible suspicion that my own arthritis (in both knees!) might be worse than his. So I could see no reason why it should make Alfred spontaneously sink to the ground; since he had been assaulted, it was much more reasonable to suppose he was on the ground because he had been punched. I couldn't then explain why his head showed so little evidence of impact, and I can't now. But, having more witness statements, I noticed that someone reported that Alfred had been wearing a thick scarf which had fallen before him and I wondered if his fall had been softened a little by the scarf on the ground. How the pathologist longs for pictures of the scene. But where there is a shred of hope that life can be preserved, nobody thinks of the forensic evidence which might be necessary after death. If anyone had recorded the incident on their phone, they, unfortunately, did not come forward.

In court, Alfred's young assailants pleaded not guilty, now claiming that they had been forced to hit Alfred in self-defence. All they had done was simply approach his son for a cigarette and he had assaulted them.

Their argument did not wash with the jury: the prosecution had too many witnesses who confirmed that the youths were the aggressors. They were found guilty of murder and sentenced to life imprisonment.

Alfred's decision to fight with the three of them had been noble but foolhardy: it showed a failure to recognize that his strength and fighting skills had declined with age. But every so often I have the strange feeling that I know the deceased. Not in life, of course, but through the autobiography written in their body. And that story is a function of the personality at its centre. I believe I liked Alfred Hoop. I suspected that his decision to fight with the three bullies to protect his son was so entirely in character that he would have done so whatever his age or medical condition. His death was probably, as so often, a product of his own unique character.

16

I had finished with Alfred Hoop and was lingering in the post-mortem room, chatting to a mortuary assistant, when I realized that one of the police officers was still there.

'Doc, I've got a bit of a tricky situation on my hands,' he began awkwardly. 'I know you don't usually do routine coronial cases, but I was just wondering . . . while you're here . . .'

I raised my eyebrows.

'I've taken the liberty of asking the coroner's office and they say you can crack on . . . if you're up for it. You'd have to give them a ring when you're finished . . .'

Of course, I wanted to go home, like everyone else, but the detective sergeant's embarrassment halted me. After a sudden, unexplained death, where the police are confident that the cause is natural, that cause must be ascertained. A specialist forensic pathologist is not necessary for this, a generalist will do (they cost less!), and the post-mortem report goes only to the coroner, not to the police. However, if there is anything suspicious about a death, the police call us. And now this detective was asking a forensic specialist to carry out a coronial post-mortem.

I studied his face, which had reddened. 'Tell me more.'

Dulcie MacMillan was sixty-seven years old. She was a busy, working artist, a portrait painter by day, but she very often spent nights in the West End, painting or repainting scenery for theatres. When she very uncharacteristically did not show up for work, her colleagues contacted the police, who broke into her house and found her on the floor.

'Look, Doc,' the detective said defensively, as if I'd been arguing with him. 'The place was a mess, but you'd expect that, she was an artist. There were paintings stacked up against the walls, old coffee cups all over the place and the floor looked as if it hadn't seen a Hoover since 1969.'

'No sign of a break-in?'

'None at all. I just thought: she's not a good housekeeper, she's quite old and she's dropped down dead.'

I nodded. 'So, no pictures, no forensics?'

'Nothing. Just shipped her off for a coroner's post-mortem, informed her niece and thought that was it.'

'What's changed your mind?'

'Her friend phoned. And a neighbour, too. Apparently, some blokes called on her last week offering to cut some branches off a tree in front of the house. And she said, no thanks. A few days later, another lot appear, offering to mend something or other. She sends them on their way, but she finds something outside her house, some lines drawn in chalk on the gatepost, which she takes to be one of those signs these people leave for each other. So she rubs out the lines. A few days later they've been redrawn. Told the neighbour she thought she was being targeted . . . and next thing, she's dead.'

'Does the neighbour think she would have let them into the house?'

'She would have opened the door, apparently, and there's no chain on it. I decided I should take another look at the mess. Went back. Niece had been in and already cleared up.'

He looked desperate.

'Doc, I wouldn't normally ask, but I've been lying awake at

night, worrying about this one. I'll be in a lot of trouble if you find someone knocked her on the head after all.'

'Right,' I said. 'Let's put your mind at rest. I'll ask the staff to bring her in.'

His face folded with relief.

'Oh, thanks, Doc.'

While the mortuary staff clanged about, I asked: 'Do we know anything about Dulcie's medical history?'

'Generally very healthy. But the niece said they'd had a curry together and it gave the old girl terrible heartburn. It was so bad she rang into work sick and the niece wondered if that was a bad sign.'

'When did they have this curry?'

He thought hard.

'Let's see. When I broke the news to her, the niece said: "I saw her only a week ago."'

By now Dulcie was arriving.

'See, Doc, it was because of the niece . . .' The detective was still sounding defensive. 'I thought the old girl must have had a serious stomach problem. And I mean, I saw there was a lot of Alka-Seltzer lying around her house.'

The sheet covering her was removed and Dulcie's body was revealed.

She was a small, plump woman. Her thick grey hair was cut in a bob. For a moment, a raised patch on the skin of one inner wrist looked suspicious. Until it lifted easily. Paint. Probably Burnt Sienna. And I found Cobalt Blue nestling under the fingernails of her right hand. I examined her closely for any wounds or bruises, but there were none.

'No signs of violence,' I said. 'And definitely no head injury.'

The detective sergeant grinned happily.

I picked up my scalpel. 'Let's take a look inside her.'

Dulcie's body made no attempt to hide her cause of death. It was visible as soon as I had cut down the midline and opened her up.

'Blimey!' said the detective. 'What's that thing doing in there?'

Where her heart should have been was a huge, indigo balloon.

'It's the pericardial sac which holds the heart. Usually, I can see straight through it, like looking through a misty window. But Dulcie's sac has filled up with blood.'

'Why, Doc?'

'Her heart muscle must have ruptured.'

I prepared to cut the thin membrane. There is only one slightly good thing about being stabbed in the heart: the knife must penetrate the pericardial sac, allowing blood from the wound it subsequently inflicts to partially drain out of the sac and so giving a chance, a very small chance, of survival. Dulcie's pericardial sac had not been cut. It was tightly distended, but still it had held the leaking blood firmly and faithfully. As it had filled, it had hugged the heart harder and harder, like a boa constrictor, until beating ceased.

'Looks really painful!' The detective winced.

'No, no, she would have been unconscious almost instantly and her death was quiet,' I assured him. 'We should all hope to go this way.'

The pericardial sac had shown resilience by retaining Dulcie's blood, but now it offered little resistance to my PM40. After death, the blood trapped inside it had clotted and the clot had formed a perfect mould around the heart. It was solid but fragile and I was able to lift it out, holding its wobbling, heart-shaped hole together very carefully.

I put the clot to one side while the detective stared at the heart that had been hidden inside it. The tear in its front wall was very prominent. It looked like a bright red rip in a piece of fabric. It was perhaps a centimetre long. After death the heart was no longer under pressure so it was not the gaping hole it must have been at the end of Dulcie's life but I could still easily poke the blunt end of my scalpel through it. Surrounding it was dead muscle. Swollen, firm – and yellow. Sorry about this, but the nearest thing I know to heart muscle in this state is egg custard.

'Alka-Seltzer wasn't going to help Dulcie,' I said.

The detective looked confused. 'I don't understand why she had a stomach problem just because her heart was on the way out.'

'She didn't. She only thought she did.'

Our ability to fool ourselves is remarkable. Dulcie was sixty-seven and overweight and I wouldn't be at all surprised to learn that one of her parents had died from a heart problem. But when she suddenly suffered from heartburn so acute that she could not go to work, she took antacid and told herself it must have been that curry. It may have crossed her mind that here was a heart attack. But she evidently preferred not to act on this suspicion. That delay had killed Dulcie, although it had at least helped the pathologist.

The heart is a ball of muscle, and when we speak of a heart attack we mean that the muscle, somewhere in the heart, has not received the oxygen it needs and has died. Technically, it is an infarction. However, if a patient dies instantly and the cause was a heart attack, there is surprisingly little evidence of this. We have to eliminate all the other explanations (of which the most obvious are stroke, pneumonia, pulmonary embolism, perforated ulcer or infection) and we do have chemical tests to help us but, if pathologists had their way, everyone would live for at least three hours after a heart attack. By then, very early ischaemic changes in the muscle have become visible, or at least palpable.

The damaged heart muscle swells and firms as the body responds to the dead tissues by sending in scavenger cells to pick up the debris. It also grows tiny new blood vessels into the area to start the process of repair. If the patient lives a week, the damaged area begins to look necrotic and turns a mottled yellow/red. At the end of a month, it is getting pale. At the end of about six months, the thin, pearly white, early scarring is easy to discern.

In Dulcie's case, she had ignored her heart attack and reached that dangerous point, about seven days later, when the scavenger cells had cleared up most of the mess but the self-repair operation had not quite started. At this stage, the damaged area of muscle is at its most vulnerable. And, it was then, when it was weakest, that Dulcie's heart muscle simply gave way. The pressure inside from the normal heartbeat stretched it beyond its limit and it ruptured. A torrent of blood would have poured into the sac, which retained it. That blood therefore squeezed the heart, preventing it from beating. The yellow/red state of the muscle surrounding the rupture dated the heart attack to about one week ago. Which fitted with the time of the so-called heartburn.

The rupture was unlucky because Dulcie, having survived the death of a part of her heart muscle, might have lived much longer. The heart is a small but noble organ which will keep on pumping despite worsening shortage of oxygen until, finally, is overwhelmed. To work properly, though, it must beat with rhythm and coordination. Lub! The two ventricular heart valves snap shut and muscle contracts to push the blood into the arteries, either towards the lungs or off around the body.

Meanwhile, the two atria at the top of the heart fill with blood. Dub! The valves that are gatekeepers to the arteries now snap shut to prevent any backflow while the valves between the atria and ventricles open and blood rushes in. Lub-Dub. Lub-Dub. Over a lifetime. About 40 million times a year. Until enough muscle cells have died to entirely disrupt this coordinated rhythm and the heart, for the first and only time, lost, confused and halting, wanders from the purpose to which it has been devoted for so many years. Death follows.

To look for the first factor in Dulcie's death, I had to find what had caused the original cardiac event a week ago and led to the rupture.

There are three arteries that supply the heart with the oxygen it needs to keep beating. One feeds the front wall of the left ventricle, one the back and side of the left ventricle and one the right ventricle. Dulcie's cells had died in the front wall of the left ventricle and so I knew at once that there must be a blockage in that artery which is called the left anterior descending.

This blockage had not caused instant death – and, actually, it is seldom that people drop down dead from a sudden, single heart event. It can happen, but myocardial infarctions, as we call heart attacks, are often a much longer, slower-evolving process than is realized. So when we are told that a man shovelling snow clutched his chest and fell to the ground, I am likely to find that parts of his heart muscle had actually been damaged and dying for days, or even weeks. The exertion of snow-shovelling had overwhelmed the ability of his narrowing artery to supply enough oxygen and so the dying cells were tipped into a final crisis. I might see further evidence of a number of heart attacks over a number of years, unknown to, or at least unreported by, the deceased. I have seen hearts which are almost covered in the white scars of dead muscle and wondered how it was possible for the deceased to have stayed alive so long.

If the carotid arteries which feed the brain become blocked, the result is probably an acute stroke or, at the other end of the temporal spectrum, vascular dementia. If an elderly person cannot walk without severe pain, arthritis is not necessarily the problem: cramps and immobility may be caused by narrowed leg arteries. But most prone of all to narrowing are the arteries which feed the heart, the coronary arteries, and this is certainly the main killer of the British in general but especially men in late middle age. Significantly fewer women are affected because they have some natural protection until they are past childbearing age. At menopause, changes in hormone levels mean that they start to catch up and, within a decade or two, when they are in their sixties or seventies, coronary heart disease is killing as many women as men.

Disease in the coronary arteries – known as coronary heart disease or ischaemic heart disease – is the world's leading cause of death, and the problem is particularly acute in Western societies. Rates are significantly lower in Japan than in other developed countries – but when the Japanese migrate to the USA, their rate shoots up, indicating the importance of diet as well as genetics to the condition.

How do arteries become blocked? The master criminal is cholesterol, which is a fat, or lipid, that is essential for making many crucial chemicals in our bodies. It also maintains the walls of our cells. Because it is essential, mankind is programmed to enjoy foods that contain these fats. The busy liver converts fat to cholesterol and releases it into the bloodstream so that it can circulate to all the cells that need it. Of course, fats are usually insoluble, but cholesterol teams up with a protein and, for about seven hours after a fatty meal, bubble-like structures called micelles, consisting of fat, salts and protein, are transported around the body. If more fat has been consumed than the body needs, the fatty bubbles tend to linger longer in the circulating blood.

The inner surface of arteries is very thin and transparent, like clingfilm. The circulating fat bubbles leak under this, against the wall of the artery. Here they form lumps and bumps of fatty gunge, called atheroma. The word 'atheroma' is Greek for porridge, and that is exactly what it looks like. As it spreads along the artery wall the larger lumps of porridge are called plaques.

Plaque is easy to see through the artery's gossamer-thin inner lining. It is usually mottled white and yellow; its exact yellowness depends on its age and fat content. If it hasn't been there long, it is squidgy to touch. But over time it might calcify, a process which covers it with something like a thin layer of ice, the sort that children like to stamp on after a very light frost. When people talk about 'furred up' arteries you might imagine the inside of a kettle, but that is not at all how plaque looks. It is more like pale butter with a thin, whiteish layer of crusty icing on top.

A healthy artery is an extremely flexible tube which I can bend with very little effort. It is far easier to wrap around my hand than an electric cable. In fact – and here we are, unfortunately, back to food analogies – it resembles spaghetti cooked *al dente*.

Most arteries are whiteish, although the mighty aorta, the chief artery that leads directly from the heart, is quite distinctively yellow. However, diseased arteries do tend to become more yellow as they grow old and stiffen. We speak of 'hardening of the arteries', and my first teacher in forensic pathology used to say that you can tell the condition of an artery just by listening carefully as you cut it. And it's true that you can often hear an artery crackle because it has become so stiff and calcified. By that stage, it sounds like dried spaghetti just out of the packet. A thorough post-mortem should involve all of the five senses, so I agree that it is worth listening to arteries – but I also concentrate on how they feel.

'You're not looking!' people have exclaimed during post-mortems as I close my eyes and feel my way along an artery. But to me, touch can be as important as sight or hearing. Knowing how healthy body parts feel makes problems easy to detect. In the case of arteries, I can determine where the problems lie by the feel of tell-tale lumps or areas of sudden stiffness.

'I won't have to go far to find the blockage,' I told the detective.

In the past we used special, small scissors to snip along the artery, but that carries a risk. You can easily push any clot that might be plugging it right out of the way. So, these days, we cut across the vessel from side to side at 2-mm or even 1-mm intervals. The left anterior descending is the West's most commonly blocked coronary artery, and now I carefully felt and sliced my way along Dulcie's, starting at the aorta. And with each cut came the light crackle I associate with breakfast cereals.

When atheroma is first deposited – a process which in Dulcie's case I would say had started many years ago – it settles just beneath the artery's inner lining of cells and is neatly contained there. Perhaps for a lifetime but, more likely, until the plaque expands. Sometimes plaques build only in patches. It is easily possible to have an entirely clear artery with a blockage in just one place, although this can be fatal because a chain is only as strong as its weakest link and an artery only as clear as its narrowest point. And that narrow place tends to be where blood flow is turbulent and the lining is more battered – just as the confluence of two rivers creates choppy waters and weaker banks.

The big aorta bends upwards and backwards over the heart and the bronchus of the left lung. It then hugs the front of the spine as it heads south, feeding the smaller arteries which in turn feed the abdominal organs. The earliest sites of plaque in young adult life – and the sites of the most serious plaque in late adult life – can be found where these smaller arteries branch off from the aorta. The bottom of the spine, where the aorta splits in two to make the iliac arteries, supplying blood to each leg, is another key area for plaque formation. And the femoral arterial system of the upper legs is so complex that there is a lot of turbulence: plaque can be found in many places here.

So the main sites for the build-up of atheroma are the aorta and those vessels running from it which supply the gut, kidneys, legs, heart and brain. I seldom see it anywhere else – the arms, for instance, generally stay clear. And veins simply do not get this build-up of plaque, presumably because the pressure here is much lower.

As plaque expands, it sometimes spreads into and damages the middle layer of the artery's wall. This is elastic muscle and it is structurally crucial. Subjected to the constant cycle of pressure–relax as the heart pumps, this layer of wall can become seriously weakened by plaque. Once this happens, it will no longer return to its normal size and shape after each pulse. The stretch remains and the artery dilates like a long, thin party balloon. This is an aneurysm. And, like a party balloon, if it is blown up too much, it can burst. If this happens, blood will pour into the abdomen, often leading to rapid death.

Plaque is more likely to build up on the inside of the artery wall. The inner lining holding it starts to bulge inwards and, of course, this narrows the passage available for blood to flow through. Here is the start of heart disease – but, initially, without symptoms. The problem is hidden. Later, there might be increased breathlessness walking uphill, or the unpleasant tightening pain in the chest of angina, or perhaps cramps in the legs or periods of dizziness. I bet Dulcie was familiar with some of these symptoms. We know she had angina but had decided it was heartburn. And then completely ignored the problem.

With plaque narrowing the artery, the blood must squeeze through a smaller channel and so further turbulence is inevitable. The very thin lining of the artery is increasingly battered and, if it then ruptures, the atheroma it was covering and containing is now released.

Two things will happen.

First, lumps of fatty gunge will whizz away in the bloodstream, probably blocking tiny arteries further along and so cutting off oxygen to whatever part of the body they supply. Second, the more solid atheroma beneath is exposed as the lining is ripped off. The body immediately seals this and the sealing process is topped by layers of blood clot.

The clotting system is not just highly efficient but so enthusiastic that it can sometimes make too much clot. Not a problem if you cut your finger, but a potential disaster inside a small artery. And so the clot, in sorting out one problem, may actually cause a much more serious one. The artery may block either right here or perhaps further downstream if the clot, too, is pushed along by blood.

Eventually blockages, if they are severe enough, can cause

the death of so much heart muscle that the heart's efficiency is affected or its rhythm disturbed. Or it is stopped altogether.

About a centimetre from the aorta, Dulcie's build-up of plaque was a firm lump under my fingers, like a small snake that had swallowed a rat. Cutting through it showed that the top of the plaque had sheared away and a blood clot had formed. The clot completely plugged the artery. It was a rich, glistening, rusty red. It was as easy to see and feel as a large blob of jam, but it was so firm that it could be squeezed out of the artery like toothpaste.

When I examined the other two coronary arteries, I found that this was by far the worst area of three very diseased vessels. If Dulcie had gone to the doctor with her heartburn, a simple ECG would have shown a problem in her coronary arteries and a cardiac specialist might have decided to put metal stents in to reopen them. Or a surgeon might have decided to bypass them all.

But does really serious atheroma such as this bring about certain death? As in the case of David Kelly, and many, many others I have seen, we can never make that assumption. Almost everyone in Western society over the age of fifty – perhaps over forty – does have a degree of atheroma. It may be minimal for some, but they are a small minority. Indeed, atheroma is so ubiquitous that, in those rare instances where I find that the deceased's arteries are completely clear, I immediately start looking for a malignancy. It seems that cancer and coronary heart disease can be mutually exclusive. Perhaps for genetic reasons. Or because some tumours are so hypermetabolic that they break down any fat they can find.

Coronary atheroma is not always fatal and, much more commonly, it just causes the heart muscle to work less efficiently. Or, as we say, to fail. Heart failure sounds as though it must be synonymous with death, but actually it is a medical condition many people live with for a long time. If she had gone to the doctor, Dulcie could have been one of them. It simply means that your heart does not have the capacity for all you may require of it, whether that is as little as walking up two steps to your front door or as demanding as a marathon. So perhaps we all have a degree of heart failure, from middle age onwards, anyway.

However, we are prone to telling ourselves we could get fit if we really wanted to. Acknowledging that our hearts are beginning to fail would mean changing our diet and lifestyle and starting a new relationship with our own mortality. Only a very few of us do that spontaneously, and Dulcie certainly did not. Although I was pretty sure that she had made one nod at mortality: she had, perhaps quite recently, given up smoking.

The plaques in her blood vessels and the way her lungs were covered in tiny bubbles told me that she had been a long-term smoker – even though, tellingly, her fingers were not now stained by nicotine. However, her teeth retained that ochre hue which no hygienist could polish away.

Heart health is down to the usual mix of genes, luck and lifestyle choices. And, of these, the most significant factor is lifestyle. However, there are known to be at least 500 different genes that raise cholesterol. The members of one family may all carry the same gene and all have an exceptionally high level of cholesterol without knowing it – until someone dies unnaturally early. There are tragic cases of even adolescents dying suddenly and apparently without cause, until their arterial plaques are noted and a sibling's cholesterol is found to be many times higher than any norm.

But not all genes are bad. In a fifteen-year study in

Mississippi, scientists targeted members of the population who had a gene which was believed to lower levels of that 'bad' fat, Low Density Lipoprotein, or LDL. All participants were aged between forty-five and sixty-four. The gene was found to reduce coronary heart disease by an astonishing 88 per cent. And this despite the fact that more than half of the participants had high blood pressure, a third smoked and about a fifth had diabetes – all significant risk factors. The scientists who carried out the study say that the gene reduced LDL levels only by 28 per cent but this seemed to cause a disproportionate fall in coronary heart disease. Another gene, which cut LDL levels by 15 per cent, was found to result in a 50 per cent reduction in coronary heart disease. So the scientists involved speculated that just a small reduction in 'bad' fat *over a lifetime* can have a major effect. They went one step further and suggested that their results added some support to a widely held theory: that the build-up of plaque starts early in life, even if its effects are not felt until much later. Based on my own experience examining people of all ages, I, personally, do not think the rot sets in until middle age.

There are many risk factors for cardiovascular problems that no one can change. Men are generally much more at risk. So are shorter people, for reasons which are not understood. In some parts of the world, particularly Asia, whole populations may be genetically predisposed. The incidence of cardiovascular problems in the UK is certainly higher among those on low incomes or those who live in areas of social deprivation. Diabetics are almost guaranteed to produce more atheroma, and even the young can suffer the effects of this if they do not take the trouble to control their condition carefully. Many kidney and certain liver problems can affect the cardiovascular system. Babies in the womb who experience some oxygen shortage (perhaps the mother has pre-eclampsia or is obese or just catches an infection at the wrong time) are also strongly suspected of suffering much later on in life from cardiovascular disease, a suspicion ignited by the long-term studies into those who were in the womb during the 1918 'flu pandemic. Living near busy roads may increase risk: air pollution has been found to have a significant effect on heart health, but it is also possible that the constant low level of stress produced by noise affects blood pressure. Finally, depression and post-traumatic stress disorder are also both recognized risk factors.

Happily, there are some risks we can manage, at least to some extent.

Anger can exacerbate an existing, silent heart problem. And so does stress, especially when associated with long working hours, a poor diet and broken sleep patterns. No smoker needs me to say this: cigarettes cause heart disease. But I, for one, sometimes need reminding that more than five units of alcohol in a day or fourteen in a week is associated with an increase in blood pressure and weight. Both these are major risk factors and can be lowered with regular exercise, which also raises the 'good' lipids in blood. We could all, in our food-rich Western society, benefit from taking a long, hard look at our diets and reviewing not just calorie content but the composition of those calories.

I wish I always followed my own advice. It is easy to understand that young people place themselves at risk with dangerous or excessive behaviour because they are oblivious to the possible consequences. It is harder to understand why the rest of us, people like me and like Dulcie, knowingly risk our heart health. I conclude that this refusal to face such facts is part of the human condition. Most of us know very well the risks of our lifestyle, but the majority of us find this information easy to ignore. For instance, despite considerable health education efforts, the percentage of the population eating five portions of fruit or vegetables a day has barely increased, if at all, since the five-a-day mantra was introduced more than ten years ago: in some demographics, it has gone down. Because, for now, our hearts keep on beating and, if our arteries complain, we can't hear them. It is only when we encounter one of the greatest risk factors of all that some of us begin to regret a lifetime of health complacency. That factor is age.

I completed Dulcie's post-mortem and the detective sergeant thanked me profusely.

'I'm glad I've put your mind at rest,' I said.

'Except, you haven't, Doc.'

I raised my eyebrows. 'She really did die of natural causes, I assure you.'

'I mean all that talk about arteries getting narrowed and no one really knowing until it's too late. I've been wondering about my own diet. And I used to be a smoker. I mean, I wish I could start again from today and do it right this time. So is there anything I can do now to clean up the mess which I've got building up in my arteries?'

'Sorry,' I said. 'The answer's probably no. A change of lifestyle could slow down or maybe even prevent further narrowing but, unfortunately, when it comes to the health of the cardiovascular system, there are no second chances.'

His face fell. Wisdom comes too late. As I, for one, know all too well.

17

I prefer not to think my memory is failing. However, I recognize that sometimes it is slower than it used to be to retrieve information. And sometimes it makes wrong retrievals. That flypast of Concorde and the Red Arrows when I was taking my A-levels which I described so breathlessly earlier in this book? I remember it as though it were yesterday. Except, subsequent research has told me it never happened. Concorde landed at Heathrow for the first time in 1970 and that is surely the occasion I recalled, but my memory inserted the Red Arrows. They were not there. I now find that it was many years afterwards that Concorde and the Red Arrows flew together and it may not have been until 2002 that I actually witnessed this, when there was a flypast over London for the Queen's Golden Jubilee.

Knowing my memory is playing that kind of trick on me feels uncomfortable. Of course, I can explain it away as a rare error. I prefer not to entertain the possibility that soon errors will become less rare. But it is less easy to shrug off a minor accident I had soon after I started to write this book.

I keep hives of bees: for fascination, relaxation and, most of all, lovely stuff to spread on toast. In the summer, as they have a habit of doing on warm, sunny days, they swarmed. This is their way of reproducing. Fortunately, this queen and her followers didn't go far. In a tree near the hive, I found a furry, drooping, wriggling blob of buzzing, vibrating potential honey dripping from a branch about eight feet up. That's an easy one for a beekeeper. Step one: ladder. Step two: cardboard box. Step three: a quick shake of the branch. Step four: new hive. Job done.

Steps one and two were successfully completed, but there are then some minutes missing from my life. I'm not sure how many. They passed between step three above and the moment I opened my eyes and found the paramedic leaning over me. I later estimated that I had been unconscious for about ten minutes. I had no idea that, after I had reached for the swarm with my box, the ladder collapsed. That my wife had found me lying on the ground with 30,000 angry bees around me. That she had called 999 while yelling for help from a neighbour. That my breathing had been, for a short time, the agonal type my wife, as a doctor, associated with impending death (laboured, gasping and irregular). That the ambulance had drawn up with its siren blaring. That the paramedics had carried out tests and performed an ECG.

I knew none of this, and those minutes are simply lost. If I had died instead of being knocked unconscious, I would have had no knowledge that I was dying. Perhaps that is how death can be. Like falling from a ladder. A painless, unexperienced event, simply the sudden arrival of – nothing. In which case, death is nothing to be feared.

Later that day I returned home from the local A&E with a small fracture in a transverse process (the spikes which stick out at the side of the spine) of a lumbar vertebra, a fading headache and a very red face. How could I have been so stupid as to stretch further than the ladder allowed? Had I assumed that I was still as slim and flexible as I had been twenty years ago? Was the whole accident a failure on my part to recognize that I am ageing? And how often in the post-mortem room have I noticed that this failure is much more dangerous than ageing itself?

I did recover, and quite quickly, but there was another unexpected consequence of my visit to the emergency department.

I was given a routine CT trauma scan while I was there.

The doctor looked at the scan and then said: 'Did you know about your liver?'

At that time, there were no words more calculated to strike horror into my heart than these. Let others dread accidents, heart attacks or even homicide; for me, it was not sudden death but cirrhosis which held terror. I did not want to live with the long-term misery of a chronically damaged liver.

You might think my fear could easily be managed by not drinking alcohol. Of course, I would agree with you. But at the time of my ladder escapade, during the long Covid lockdown summer of 2020, I will admit to an extraordinary escalation in my alcohol use.

I worked all day but tried to take the evenings off. When the day's busyness was over, when the dogs were walked, when the supper was cooking, well, then I liked to pour myself a drink. My predilection for whisky and soda dates back to holidays with my father-in-law on the Isle of Man: as a former colonial, he could be counted on to settle down to one every evening and, when we stayed there, so did I. That is when I started to associate that drink with a good life, well lived. With the quiet of the declining day. With reward for hard work finished. With pleasure, relaxation and good humour.

So each evening now, I poured myself one drink. Did I measure it? Of course not. There's a line, part of its design, on the glass I drink from, and that's where I stopped pouring. I sometimes wondered how many shots were below the line. Certainly, more than one. I decided it must be two.

I drank slowly. I relaxed. And when I finished . . . I often poured another. I was probably reading, talking or watching TV, but a glass was usually in my hand. During the evening meal, I'd consume my half of a bottle of wine . . . actually, sometimes a bit more than my half.

It was a long time before I started doing the maths and, even then, in true drinker fashion, I wasn't honest with myself. So, a double whisky twice, that's four units. And half a bottle of wine, that's five. A total of nine units a night. I was doing this every night of the week. Nine units, seven nights a week . . . that's . . . no, surely not. Every drinker is capable of claiming that there are only four days in a week. But, trying to be strictly honest, I admitted to myself that I was consuming sixty-three units a week, more than four times the recommended maximum and with no days off to rest my liver.

I knew I had to change. I resolved to give up drinking for at least a week. But that evening, at 7 p.m., I was miserable. And anyway, how was my alcohol consumption having any real effect? The whiskies were something to enjoy at home, so driving wasn't an issue. I certainly wasn't falling around or starting any fights. I was no risk to myself or others and I was always sober and ready for work in the morning. Where was the harm? I ended my suffering and reached for the bottle.

One night I heard a voice muttering – or was it actually raised? – during the TV news. Was it my voice? Expressing opinions I might normally not have articulated. Not so strongly, anyway. Afterwards, I couldn't quite remember if I had said anything out loud or only thought it. I asked my wife. Apparently, I'd said it out loud.

I didn't always sleep well and there were mornings when I woke up with my mind a little clouded, wishing I had at least not drunk the wine. But without a ritual drink in the evening, I didn't get that feeling of relaxation and reward that was such an important part of my wind-down after a working day – actually, after any day. For me, drink didn't feel destructive, it felt life-enhancing. There are so many different drinking patterns according to class, financial status and age. Welcome to my elderly professional's landscape of entirely socially acceptable home drinking. And we were in lockdown. I told myself that everyone was doing it.

Lockdown temporarily eased and I spent some time with older relatives and didn't consume a drop for a few days. Since I was away from home, no 7 p.m. bell rang inside my head. Abstinence made me feel sharper, brighter. So well, in fact, that I resolved that, once back, I would break my whisky habit. And after making this resolution, I decided to be wholly honest. I had been honest before, but that had been a drinker's honesty. Now I was stopping, so I could tell the truth, the whole truth.

I admitted that I had frequently consumed more than two double whiskies; in fact, I had generally been consuming three. So, last week and much of the summer, the man I was then had been drinking a hideous total of not sixty-three units a week but seventy-seven. That man appalled me. Every night, he was consuming almost the maximum recommended for an entire week. I really didn't want to know him any more, no matter how much he thought he deserved his evening tipple.

But he was soon back.

I can't remember if my resolve was weakened by the sight of my wife sipping a gin and tonic in the garden on a long, warm summer's evening or the incredible discounts

Sainsbury's were offering on my favourite whisky. It wasn't long before I was trying to get empty bottles in the recycling before my wife noticed them and even surreptitiously topping up my glass if she left the room for a few moments. One night I found myself asking a terrible question. Was I addicted?

A widely used definition of addiction is that, through drink or drug dependency, life has become unmanageable. I decided that certainly wasn't me. Another definition is that, until the substance is consumed, you don't feel completely normal: in other words, there is no beneficial 'high' associated with consumption but without it there is an absence and a 'low'. Filling that absence merely restores perceived normality. I knew that could be me. Now when have I been in this bind before? Ah yes, all those years I tried to give up smoking.

I was fully aware of the dangers of cigarettes; after all, I routinely examined diseased lungs and overworked hearts. I frequently woke up in the morning determined that today would be the day I would change. I reasoned with myself, I set deadlines, my brain and my habit made deals, I admonished myself frequently and stopped for days, weeks or even months . . . but I always started smoking again. Until one day, in midlife, I really knew I wanted to stop this time. Really. And, quite simply, I did.

And now, I reasoned, it was time, in the same way, to give up drinking. I had admitted to myself the extent of the problem, I really wanted to stop and I did not want to enter the post-pandemic world, which everyone hoped might be approaching, with an alcohol dependency.

I tried. But I could not shake my lockdown habit. My consumption was staying stubbornly high. And now I was cross.

I began to dislike myself. It seemed that not me but my whisky was deciding I would drink it. The loss of control was downright scary and quite shameful.

So when I fell off the ladder and was informed by the doctor that the scan had shown something was wrong with my liver, I experienced a moment of terror and, in that moment, a screen I had somehow been placing between me and the truth suddenly lifted.

Of course there was something wrong with my liver! I knew very well that the measure in that glass wasn't giving me double whiskies. I checked. Yup. It was giving me more like quadruples. That's twelve units a night in three glasses of whisky, plus five units of wine, that's seventeen units a night, *which was 119 units a week*. I can't pretend I woke up each morning with a clear mind, but I had no banging headache, as one might expect. Which meant that my liver was becoming habituated to dealing with this deluge of alcohol. And, believe me, that really is not a good sign, especially if the drinker is foolish enough to have no alcohol-free days for the liver to repair itself. And this drinker was that foolish.

I thought of all the livers I had seen with the unmistakable fattiness of foie gras, of the livers that were enlarged and pale like a huge bowl of proven but uncooked dough. Greasy dough. Ugh. And now the doctor was going to tell me that my liver was one of those. Fatty. And perhaps enlarged.

Oh, the hypocrisy. When I looked in the mirror, I saw a man who believes in Western medicine and values vaccination and all the other remarkable advances in the prevention and treatment of disease. But I also saw a man who chooses to ignore the scientific evidence that he is damaging his body and endangering his health by drinking so much. I wasn't sure how any sentient human being could do this and I determined then and there, lying in a curtained cubicle in A&E, to stop.

'What's wrong with my liver?' I asked the doctor, trying to hide my panic.

'You've got a cyst on it,' he said.

I felt relief wash all over me. It was like sinking into a warm bath.

'Oh, just a cyst!' I said happily. Whatever else causes cysts, it isn't alcohol.

'Maybe you'll want to look into that?' he suggested.

I was almost laughing now.

'No, no, if it's just a cyst . . . I was probably born with it!'

I arrived home feeling far happier than a man who had just fallen off a ladder should. Of course, I needed a drink. That night, my hand hovered over the whisky. For a whole second. It was usually a reward, but after a day like this one, it was compensation. I promised myself that I would finish the bottle but buy no more. This I adhered to for a couple of weeks. Until there was another special offer on my favourite brand.

'Can't you just drink in moderation?' asked my wife, a woman who is capable of making a gin and tonic last all evening.

I tried, and I couldn't. So there was only one thing to do, and that was give up completely.

I didn't.

Then a letter arrived from the hospital. It called me for a liver scan.

Horrified, I phoned at once. I really couldn't attend that appointment because I was carrying out a post-mortem. I hoped they wouldn't find me another one. Unfortunately, the clerk promised to do exactly that.

'Er . . . who says I need this appointment?' I asked.

She named the hospital's liver specialist and told me I could expect to have an ultrasound scan soon.

'Is this necessary?' I asked. 'It's only a cyst.'

She sighed and assured me that the specialist would carry out only necessary tests. I already knew that. And it didn't take me long to work out that the scan report from A&E had gone to my GP, who was far too alert. He had noticed the liver cyst and had now helpfully referred me back to the hospital.

How I dreaded this appointment. I knew there was a risk that the scan would show a very unattractive liver indeed. And, after that, there would be a consultation with the specialist, and he would ask me: 'How much do you drink?' and then possibly try to separate me from my evening companions, whisky and soda.

I did not want a scan or a specialist to do that. I wanted to do it myself.

This time, I really did stop drinking. Completely. Six weeks later, more than four kilos lighter and with a lower than usual blood pressure, I went to the liver clinic and saw my healthy liver on the screen. It had taken advantage of my abstinence and carried out necessary repairs. As for the cysts, there were three of them. We joked about their possible causes – the specialist for fun, me from anxiety. All those infections, those worms that I'd learned about . . .

I said: 'Er . . . they're not hydatid cysts, I hope.'

'I've only ever seen them in farmers. Do you keep livestock?'

'No.'

'Relax. Your cysts are congenital and pose no threat.'

If it crossed my mind that evening to pour myself a celebratory drink, the thought was a fleeting one. Looking back on my daily consumption, it is clear to me that, although I had insisted I felt fine during my period of excess, I really had not felt so very well. The effects of alcohol have a long tail, and that tail reaches into the next morning. My productivity was probably down by at least 10 per cent and, really, I did not enjoy the start of the day. Of course, I could have the odd glass of wine now if I want to – I recognize how pleasantly one glass adds an extra dimension to a meal – but I prefer not to open myself to alcohol's insidious properties again.

My age group's propensity to reward ourselves with alcohol is reflected in the numbers who die from it but, although still significant, those numbers peak in late middle age and from there start falling away. For my own cohort, another vice takes the greater harvest. It is nicotine.

Wartime Britain was a nation of smokers and, for many years afterwards, we remained so. At around the time I was born, in the early 1950s, the pioneering epidemiologist Richard Doll was drawing attention to the effects of smoking on health. This news met with immense resistance. As my lockdown drinking proved to me, knowing that something is bad for you is one thing, changing an addictive habit is another.

Why on earth did my generation take up smoking, when we were lucky enough to be the first to know all about its hazards before we even started? The answer must be that we followed the example of others. And we fell for the advertising. How well I remember that rugged man in a rugged landscape, looking into the mid-distance from his horse, cigarette, of course, a necessary part of that evocative scene. A number of actors took part in that famous campaign and they almost all died of lung cancer or chronic lung disease.

I can't blame my father for setting a bad example. Mine was a non-smoking – actually, an anti-smoking – household. But outside the home I was surrounded by people who had no intention of stopping. For all of our youth and most of our lives, the fug of smoke meant comfort, happiness, adulthood. If not at home, then on every bus or train, in every café or pub, down every street. At work, the offices and the corridors were thick with fumes, even in hospitals, and there were day rooms off the wards set aside especially for smokers.

I started smoking when I started medical school. Oh, the irony. It took me more than twenty years to kick the habit, and many others did not kick it at all. That smoking cohort is here in the nation's statistics, dying now through a wide variety of cancers, through the chronic lung conditions that smoking causes, or partially hidden behind the figures for cardiovascular disease. Over the years, one might expect smoking-related cancers to lose their place as leading causes of death because fewer people smoke, especially younger people. But, although smoking is now at very low levels in the developed world, this is not true elsewhere. People who have immigrated to this country often hang on to their habit, as UK-born smokers did for many years, and this is likely to be reflected in the death statistics for some time to come.

Richard Doll's words on this subject form part of a memorial to him:

Death in old age is inevitable, but death before old age is not. In previous centuries 70 years used to be regarded as humanity's allotted span of life, and only about one in five lived to such an age. Nowadays, however, for non-smokers in Western countries, the situation is reversed: only about one in five will die before 70, and the non-smoker death rates are still decreasing, offering the promise, at least in developed countries, of a world where death before 70 is uncommon. For this promise to be properly realised, ways must be found to limit the vast damage that is now being done by tobacco and to bring home, not only to the many millions of people in developed countries but also the far larger populations elsewhere, the extent to which those who continue to smoke are shortening their expectation of life by so doing.

My own life confirms the words of the great epidemiologist. In the year of my birth, life expectancy was an average of 69.17 years, a bit more for a woman, a bit less for a man. I haven't reached that age yet, so there is still a possibility that I might drop dead when I am 69.17 (21 November, 2022, since you ask). However, by the time I had negotiated my way around life's hazards, given up smoking and arrived at my current age of sixty-eight, my life expectancy had shot up to a much more cheering eighty-three years of age.

I have embraced life's heart hazards, smoking too long and drinking too much, but there is one risk factor I have been very lucky to avoid. It is clinically recognized but little understood, and it tends to affect older members of the community – although it may have a particular relevance to anyone isolated for long periods during the pandemic lockdowns. That factor is loneliness. Most of us can acknowledge the importance of family and friends in our lives: certainly, without them, everything in my world would be smaller. But a characteristic of my age group is that life's changes and losses mean that by now many are entirely alone.

Given the mysterious but proven link between coronary heart disease and loneliness, I can speculate, but only speculate, that loneliness was the killer in one of my earliest cases. After more than 23,000 post-mortems I might be expected to have forgotten a lot of them. But not this one.

In 1990, I was a keen young pathologist, eager to put many, many years of study and training into practice. I rushed off whenever the phone rang, and one afternoon it called me to a Surrey mortuary. The night before, there had been a strong gale and, as I left the city behind me, I noticed that boughs from fallen trees had been cut up and heaved to the side of the road. I little guessed that the gale was the reason for my call.

A coroner's officer and just one very junior police constable were waiting for me at the mortuary, and around them was an assortment of boxes and plastic sacks. There were none of the usual sealed exhibit bags and this, as well as the paucity of police officers, told me that the after-effects of the gale were taking up resources and that someone had made a decision: neither the deceased nor this case was very important.

The coroner's officer explained that a tree which had fallen in the high wind had revealed human bones at its base. The wood was close to Dorking but seldom, if ever, visited: it had once been part of a grand landscape and immense gardens, but all that had crumbled now and the area where the body was found was extremely overgrown. There had only been someone onsite today to survey the tree damage after the previous night's gale.

My first reaction was a certain cynicism because pathologists are always being presented with bones. Reluctantly, by builders, who know that if this turns out to be a Viking all work will stop while the archaeologists move in. Or enthusiastically by DIYers digging the foundations for a house extension who think they might be hot on the trail of a murder mystery. Nearly always, bones that are found in this way turn out to be animal bones. In this case, however, the coroner's officer assured me that the first find had been a human skull, so there could be no mistake.

A speedy glance through the pictures handed to me by the constable showed me a skull on the woodland floor and, scattered nearby, a few long bones. A femur, the large bone in the thigh, was the most obvious, but there were others.

Finally, I could see clothes, although these were barely distinguishable from the landscape. The police had excavated carefully at first but had then just put everything they found into the bags and boxes for me to sort out.

I studied the pictures further. Had the body actually been there before the tree grew over them? I decided this was probably not the case. The tree had fallen up the steep slope it grew on and had caused a slight landfall: it was the landfall that had exposed the body.

One glance at the boxes, one sniff of their earthy smell, told me that this skeleton had been *in situ* for a very long time. I now tried to establish from the pictures whether the body had been buried in a shallow grave. Perhaps. But not necessarily. It was also possible that the deceased had died here, near the tree, and been gradually covered, over the years, by leaf litter and other woodland debris. The uprooting of one tree causes immense structural and ecological disturbance to the woodland floor and so it would be very hard to distinguish a dug area from a disturbed area.

I decided to deal with the artefacts first. Everything in the bags was bunched and scrunched, and the way it was encrusted with soil confirmed that it had been bunched and scrunched in one place for a long time.

There was a tweedy pair of trousers which had probably been green once. A dark, single-breasted jacket had become almost separated from its lining in places, but the arm bones were still within one sleeve.

'Urrrrgh,' said the young constable. 'That's what you see in horror films.'

I carefully disentangled the jacket from the bone. There was no hand at the end of it. Rats or mice usually make short work of both hands and feet if they are exposed.

A disintegrating woollen jumper that was now the colour of soil might have been fawn once. There was no label in it but beneath it was a wallet containing some coins, the latest dated 1975. Two keys on a Double Diamond fob. A tobacco tin and matches. Two strong, brown lace-up shoes, one of which had been found with the trousers, as if there were a body still inside, while the other was a few feet away, nearer the woodland surface. Neither had laces. But both contained the small bones of the feet inside what remained of the socks.

All this told us that the deceased was probably a man and, from the clothing and effects, it seemed to me that he was probably a man in late middle age or older when he had died. The style and preservation of the clothing indicated that here was no Tudor yeoman but someone who had been alive twenty years ago. And therefore, if the deceased had been a homicide victim, his killer may well still be around.

I felt that this man, whoever he was, had already been written off by the police. I saw it as my job, and my duty to the deceased, to establish, from this extraordinarily unprom-ising collection, whether there was any evidence of homicide. So far, there wasn't. For instance, the clothing did not show any tearing indicative of knife entry or a struggle.

However, there was one interesting and possibly very helpful feature.

Inside the trousers pocket, across the lining, was written by a neat hand in green marker pen: N HAMILTON LYTT and, beneath it, 25-3-75.

This prompted a lot of speculation from all three of us. Why would someone write their name in their pocket? And what did the date mean? Could it be the date he had died – given that 1975 was the year of the last-dated coin in his pocket? In which case, not an accident or a heart attack but either a very odd homicide or, more likely, suicide could be assumed. Although it seemed a strange thing for a suicidal person to do – write a name and date to give the police a few pointers when their skeleton was found years later.

The man's name was now assumed to be N Hamilton Lytt (for some reason, we chose to call him Neil) and the police constable was sure it would not take long to find out more about him: he rang his office at once with the information. But that did not stop the speculation.

Personally, I wondered if the strange identification indicated that Neil had suffered from dementia or some other mental health problem and that his name had been written there by a helper in case he got lost. If he had died in the late 1970s or early 1980s, then he might have come from one of the huge institutions – there were certainly a few in Surrey – which protected but sometimes also incarcerated the vulnerable. In the 1980s, there was a shift to care in the community and many inmates of these institutions found themselves in the wider world for the first time, and some could not cope at all. Had Neil been one of them?

If he was cared for, I speculated that Lytt might not be a name but an abbreviation for the name of his facility. And there was always the possibility that this was someone else's name. The deceased might have been homeless, or anyway been given clothes by the Salvation Army, and N Hamilton Lytt could have been the clothes' previous owner.

All this speculation told us how much we didn't know, and

probably wouldn't know, so I continued with my task of sorting and examining.

Most of the bones were in a box. I was sure after careful study that they were all from one individual. This is something it is important to establish and, in 1990, before the widespread use of DNA, it was a question of judgement and not scientific analysis. They certainly looked as though they had come from the same body and there were no duplicates, so this assumption seemed safe.

The bones were brown, like the soil. The forensics team had found no other bodily fragments: all but the bones had rotted or been eaten by animals. It was a shame the police had determined that this case was not important enough to consume many scarce resources. A very careful four-cubic-metre search might have yielded a lot more – or, anyway, some of the smaller bones, which could have been revealing.

We set about scrubbing the bones clean in the sink.

Neil's skull was without a lower jaw, and the upper jaw had no teeth, although I could see from the sockets that at the time of his death there had been teeth. Shoulder and arm bones were present on both sides. So were pelvic bones, as well as ten left ribs and nine right ribs. Nineteen of the twenty-four articulated vertebrae were present. We had much of a right leg but nothing of the left. There were no hands, but the small bones of the feet had been neatly retained.

I laid out the skeleton on a white sheet as though doing a jigsaw puzzle. This is a task I enjoy, and the officers watching me were fascinated. The human skeleton looks both strange and beautiful when presented in two dimensions. Neil's skeleton had a similarity to a curious but lovely tree, the ribs spreading outwards from the topmost and the line of strong vertebrae running like a trunk down the middle.

The skull seemed to confirm my instinct, borne out by the clothes, that this was the body of a man. Those ridges above the eye where our eyebrows perch, the supraorbital ridges: they are usually more prominent in males, as are the mastoid processes. Completely relying on these features to determine the sex of a skeleton is dangerous, as there can be so many variations. For instance, Afro-Caribbean women often have large supraorbital ridges. However, I was fairly sure that Neil was male: female skulls tend to be rounder and smoother in shape and slightly smaller than male skulls.

To the novice, the human skeleton appears to be just a mess of lumps, bumps, grooves and angles. But each is there for its own special reason and, if you can read bones, they are fascinating, especially if you are trying to establish whether the skeleton is male or female.

The first thing to examine was the pelvic bone, to determine the shape of the greater sciatic notch. Here the mantra is 'L' for Lucy and 'J' for Johnny. Neil was definitely a Johnny. Next, the angle at the front of the pelvis – the symphysis pubis. It was sharp like a steeple, so, again, another tick for male. And, finally, I looked down through the pelvic hole to determine its overall shape. Neil's was not an oval which would allow a baby's head to pass through but instead a neat 'O'. He was a man, all right. And by measuring the lengths of his remaining long bones on a special osteometric board and applying the standard formulae, I estimated that he had been somewhere between five foot five and five foot eight.

We re-examined pictures of the scene carefully for any more clues about his death. But there was nothing. Just dirty clothes and brown, old bones, hard to see because they were scattered and well camouflaged. The explanation for the missing bones and the scattering is, of course, predators.

And there are many. Some are large like foxes and dogs, others smaller like rats and mice, and some smaller still: the insects and bacteria which contribute so much to the vital process of returning us to the earth. Dust to dust. The large predators can and do drag body parts to the surface if they are not too deeply buried. They don't always sit down to a meal immediately – very often, to the fury of pathologists, they carry bones off and gnaw them far away – while the smaller predators are very grateful for fragments of clothing or hair to line their burrows.

Of those bones that remained, the toothmarks of mauling animals were clear, but there was nothing to indicate that Neil had met with an accident or an assassin. If he had fallen and then simply died of hypothermia, there was no way of telling that from the bones available. If he had been attacked with a knife, the perpetrator's secret had died with Neil. And then I noticed a slight swelling on one of Neil's ribs, suggesting that it had once been broken. If we found out who he was, this might indicate violence at the time of death, in which case the police might be more interested. But, after turning it this way and that, I decided that it was an old fracture – probably dating from a year or so before death. Hardly likely to indicate a cause for Neil's demise.

Judging his age was a bit more difficult. It always is, if the deceased has passed the early twenties. There was some slight arthritis in the one knee. And the teeth had all erupted. Sockets for the third molars – the wisdom teeth – were present. Most of the other teeth were just empty sockets and some had been missing in life, but the jaw had healed over. The few that were present were in poor condition, worn down and with the tell-tale eternity ring of encircling calculus near their bases.

Some osteoporosis in the bones, early arthritis, worn down teeth . . . even the tobacco tin seemed age-relevant. Putting it all together, I reckoned that Neil had been between sixty and seventy when he died.

The key question the police wanted answered was: how long had he been dead? There were all sorts of artefacts to examine. If they had been prepared to pay a matches or a tobacco expert (I'm sure there are such people), I daresay the contents of the tin Neil carried could have helped. Maybe the clothes could be dated, too. But the police were simply relying on me to answer this very difficult question.

I was sure that Neil must have been dead for at least five years for total decomposition to have taken place and for the bones found on the surface to have become so weathered. The most recent coins on him were dated 1975, which was fifteen years ago. I plumped for the midway point between these two possibilities and suggested that he had died ten years ago, in 1980. Perhaps.*

Of course, I had to give the cause of death as: Unascertained. And in my files Neil had a number, and the name of the file was BONES. I felt sure that sooner or later he would be identified. Surely, someone must have reported N Hamilton Lytt missing, and if the police combed their missing person files they would find a carer, a friend, a neighbour, a family member . . .

Time went by and the detectives who had been following up the name of N Hamilton Lytt finally reported that there was absolutely no owner of that name in the UK who had

* This case is so old and the deceased died so long ago, apparently unconnected to anyone, that I have allowed myself to break my own rule and reveal information that might identify him.

been alive in 1975. He did not exist on any list or register. And no one had reported the disappearance of a man fitting what little description we had of Neil.

To my surprise, the police then decided to invest in a three-dimensional facial reconstruction from the skull. This was extremely fashionable around that time, and it wasn't cheap. Most reconstructions were created painstakingly from clay, and some had certainly been uncannily accurate and had resulted in the identification of missing persons. But I was sceptical. They had the main part of a skull, but not the jaw, from a man who had probably died ten years ago, and only a few of his teeth. How accurate could such a reconstruction be?

Neil's image was originally sculpted, but I was supplied with a two-dimensional photo to place, electronically, over a picture of the skull. That was the end of my doubts. Here, surely, was Neil. As I faded from one image to the other, the skull beneath became visible, and so naturally did the face fit over it that the picture looked like a black-and-white snap of someone's uncle. Wearing jumper, shirt and tie, in the way older men did then, even for casual dress, Neil looked exactly like a man you must know. Not well. But whom you saw fairly often. That mild-mannered *Daily Express* reader on the train every morning, or the dog-walker you regularly exchanged a few words with, or the quiet brother who stayed with the neighbours a lot, or . . . well, in that picture I saw a real living, breathing man and not a half-skull found lying in woodland, kicked around by foxes.

I was sure that circulation of the picture would bring forward a relative or friend of Neil's.

It did not.

Neil's bones and the mysterious pocket inscription N

HAMILTON LYTT are still listed by the National Crime Agency's Missing Persons Unit. To this day, no one has stepped forward to say they knew him or to suggest who he might have been. In life, he was apparently invisible; in death, forgotten. But not by me. I have examined the body of many unidentified individuals over the years. Generally, eventually, identification comes through. One man, who was found not so far away from Neil and not so long before him, was identified by his pacemaker – each pacemaker has a serial number and it was not too difficult to track down the name of its owner and discover that this was a local man who had gone out for a walk and not come back. He had been reported missing by his wife nine months earlier.

We must assume that, in his later years at least, Neil lived an itinerant life, so his absence from a usual place did not alarm anyone. Sometimes old people are found in their homes, bodies decomposed, neighbours alerted only by the smell, because nobody noticed their absence from the world outside and no one was worried when they failed to answer the phone. In these cases, there may be a degree of decomposition which makes it impossible to confirm that death was through natural causes. So much can happen to the old or vulnerable when they are always by themselves – cruel tricksters can take advantage of weakness, no one hears when there is a call for help, and when problems feel overwhelming there may be no hand to offer support.

What led to this man's death on a lonely hillside so close to a town? What in his history resulted in the indifference of those around him? Neil was a ghost when he lived, and his death still haunts me.

18

I was called to an expensive and attractive house. It was in a busy residential area near a main road and a railway line but there was little noise here because it was set well back in a mature and well-tended garden. The drive was lined by banks of azaleas which, as this was May, were in full and fiery bloom.

The police had warned me there were two bodies, a husband and wife. On hearing this, I had immediately expected a murder-suicide. These are usually quite straightforward. If the woman is lying on the kitchen floor with a knife in her back and the man is in the living room with close-contact shotgun wounds, no one needs to consult the Vidocq Society.

However, the officer then added that the couple were very elderly, and I knew at once that we had a more complex case on our hands. Murder-suicide is for the passionate or, anyway, those who fear the diminution of love and its partner, lust. Elderly couples experience many emotions, but extreme passion is seldom one of them. They are too busy coping. Yes, we must now examine the inevitability which is old old age. Not senility. But past that tipping point from young old age to old old age. The tipping point is hard to recognize, partly because its arrival is so gradual and partly because for some people it comes late and for others surprisingly early.

Perhaps it can be defined as a loss of some, although not yet all, independence. Or as the introduction of limitation. In this cohort, many previously busy, active people find that their lives have become curtailed through physical pain, illness or a sense of fatigue that has crept up on them over the years and which makes the armchair increasingly attractive. Hobbies like gardening have gradually changed from a pleasure to a list of chores that must be reluctantly tackled – or someone else found to tackle them. Holidays, once organized and antici-pated in a carefree manner, may now only be truly relaxing if accompanied by adult offspring. Even then, holidays may gen-erate anxiety at the loss of usual routines or the possibility that something needed – a bathroom on hand, lunch, a drink before supper, a good local doctor – may not be available.

Instead of leaving stress to the young, who are busy like spiders as they spin their life's complex web, the very old are often anxious. Anxious that their needs will not be met or that their new physical and perhaps mental limitations have outstripped their abilities. People who thirty years ago were captains of industry may now find a manoeuvre as simple as changing trains a psychological and physical challenge. The chronic pain of long-term conditions or periodic short-term problems contributes to the tumble towards dependency. As children, our world got larger and larger until, from our twenties, it became all ours. Now, in old old age, our world becomes significantly smaller. We devote much of the time to managing our failing bodies. And we start to rely on others, just as when we were children.

So when the police officer warned me that we had a double death in an elderly household, I expected to walk into a tangled knot of loss, limitation and dependency. An over-grown garden, loose paving on the path, peeling paintwork, a greenhouse with algae all over the glass: these are some of the signs outside a house of old age within it.

But not here. I saw a well-kept garden, clean windows and recently painted frames. The only indication that anything could be wrong was a walking stick, leaning against the outside wall by the door.

At the house I was met and briefed by an officer. He opened the front door slowly, and I soon understood his caution. It would have been easy to trip over the body immediately inside.

'This is Mrs Mason-Grant,' he said.

The elderly woman was smartly dressed in a tweed skirt, sensible shoes and tights. She was lying face up, her feet just inside the door, her head a few yards from the first riser of the stairs. Her cardigan and blouse had been pulled away and blue ECG pads had been placed on her chest by the ambulance crew. Her tights had been cut, perhaps by the forensic medical examiner, in order to take her temperature. I was pleased, if so. I knew there would be a lot of questions about time of death.

I also took Mrs Mason-Grant's temperature. The bodies had been found at ten that morning, the FME had apparently been here soon after that time, and a forensic team had been busy all day. It was now after five.

A CSI was edging past us.

'I don't suppose you've recorded the room temperature?' I asked, expecting a blank look in reply.

From behind his mask, the man squinted at me.

'Doc!' he said. 'I went to your last crime-scene lecture at HQ and now it's the first thing I do every time.'

I raised my eyebrows. Had someone actually been listening to me?

'Even at burglaries!' he added. 'I've taken the temperature right here and beside her old man upstairs. Both of them, on the hour, every hour since we arrived.'

I felt like shaking his hand.

I had a brief look at the deceased in the hall for any obvious injuries. There were none. But even this rapid examination told me how very thin she was.

Next to her was a stout, plaid bag. Its leather handles were worn, telling of many shopping trips. Probably Mrs Mason-Grant had walked to the convenience store which I had driven past a couple of corners away. I looked inside the bag. Aha. Her morning walk was likely to be the same every day. Down the drive and round the block to buy a newspaper, some milk . . . and two bottles of vodka. I looked at the police officer and he raised his eyebrows but said nothing.

He led me into the living room. The forensics team was finishing now and, as they left, the house grew bigger and quieter.

'They couldn't find any evidence of a break-in,' the police officer told me. 'We're wondering if someone forced their way in when Mrs Mason-Grant got home, just as she unlocked the door . . .'

'There are no signs of a struggle here,' I said.

'Wait until you see upstairs.'

The living room was opulent. It had fine antique furniture and substantial curtains. It was very tidy. There was a large black-and-white photo of a long-ago wedding, probably the Mason-Grants' wedding. The groom was in uniform.

'He was in the army?'

'He's Colonel Mason-Grant, I believe,' the officer told me.

There were smaller photos on the piano. Some had the cloudiness of pictures of the long dead but a few were brighter and showed children. The Mason-Grants' children, I thought, rather than any grandchildren. All boys, and in each one the child was standing stiffly in school uniform. No huge, spontaneous smiles or muddy footballers. These boys must be grown-up by now but there were no pictures past the age of about twelve. Here was a very correct family, I thought. Had their children died? Or simply become less correct and therefore not suitable for photographs? There was no dust on the piano, but it was hard to imagine anyone actually playing it. Especially if they missed a note.

By one of the armchairs was a canterbury holding newspapers which were precisely folded to reveal a completed crossword. The *Telegraph*, the same paper that I had seen in the shopping bag. I imagined that, every day, Mrs Mason-Grant sat with her pen in the chair, which, now I looked closely, was worn at the arms. It was easy to think of her reading the paper, finishing the crossword and then dropping it into the canterbury. What drink would be on the side table? Tea? Or had the vodka perhaps been for her? And why had this routine been so abruptly ended today?

The kitchen was large enough to have a central island. It was spotlessly tidy and most of the surfaces were bare. There was no evidence of any recent cooking or eating.

Here was a well-ordered house, where habits and routines were adhered to. We went upstairs and found guest bedrooms. One was in use. The single bed was neatly made, covers turned down. A small travelling alarm clock, bright pink, sat on the bedside table ticking quietly, giving the sparse room a splash of colour. The alarm was set for 6 a.m. The other rooms clearly had not been slept in for some time. One had become the ironing room and had neat piles of laundry folded on the bed.

Then we reached the master bedroom and everything changed. The chaos was so palpable it seemed I could close my eyes and still sense it. I picked my way through the littered floor to the elderly man who lay in pyjamas, face up, in the centre of the room.

Once again, the paramedics had left their signature: blue ECG pads. Once again, I could not immediately find any injuries. Once again, I noted that here was someone very thin.

I took Colonel Mason-Grant's temperature and then looked around.

Nearby was an upturned stool. The bedclothes were tangled. There were laundry piles strewn around the floor.

'Think there's been a bit of a tussle in here?' asked the police officer hopefully. I shook my head. Yes, every surface was covered chaotically. Much but not all of the clutter was medical: tissues, bandages, scissors, sticking plaster, cream, tubes of emollient, nail files, pens, a golf trophy, some military-looking badges and, mysteriously, a small statue of the Eiffel Tower. There had been a system in this room once and then, for some reason, the system had been ignored and nothing returned to its right place. This is churn. It is a different kind of madness from the chaos intruders leave behind.

I did see, on the dressing table, a couple of empty vodka bottles. They were standing innocently surrounded by bottles of cosmetics and medicine, the way shoplifters try to mingle with the crowds.

I looked for more bottles in the bedroom but found none. Probably the two full bottles in the hall were expected and the two empty ones ready to go out. A system of sorts in this ocean of disorder. And there were two jars, one on the dressing table, the other by the bed, of dark, mucoid material. It looked like some sort of bodily waste, something the old man might spit up.

By now, possible scenarios were starting to occur to me

and I had seen enough. It was time to find out more at post-mortem. But, since it was already seven o'clock and I had finished two other post-mortems earlier that day, the detectives agreed that we should reconvene at the mortuary the following morning.

When I arrived, the staff said that Colonel and Mrs Mason-Grant were ready and waiting outside the post-mortem room. They asked who we were going to start with.

'Let's do Mrs Mason-Grant first, she's more likely to hold the key to all this,' I said as I set off in the opposite direction towards the bereavement centre. Here were, luckily, no bereaved people. Instead, the police sat, hunched over tea and peering past the broken Nice in the biscuit box for the Custard Creams.

They recapped everything they knew. The old couple had been found yesterday morning by one of their three sons: he had no key but, after knocking repeatedly, he had tried the front door and been amazed to find it was unlocked. In general, his parents greatly discouraged any impromptu visits. The order I had seen inside most of the house evidently extended to the way the couple conducted their relationships. Family members were allowed to visit only by prior arrangement, and there were not to be too many visits and no one was to stay too long. All the sons and their families knew the rules and somehow had been persuaded to abide by them very strictly.

One of the sons had tried to phone his parents at the weekend and there had been no reply. That was not unusual. But when he had phoned a second and a third time and no one had answered, he was surprised. He had alerted his brothers, who had also tried. Nothing. You might think that was sufficiently alarming for one of them, the son who lived locally, perhaps, to head straight over on Monday morning, at the latest. But he was too well trained for that. Keen to avoid annoying his parents by dropping by unannounced, he continued to phone them, and so did the others.

On Tuesday night, it was agreed between all three that they would the next day be able to justify an unauthorized visit. The nearest son was to go to the house in the morning, but not too early, in fact, at ten o'clock, by which time Mrs Mason-Grant had usually finished her shopping. But if the parents showed any displeasure at this sudden arrival, he was to withdraw immediately.

We looked at each other and munched on our biscuits.

'They must have been a scary mum and dad,' one of the detectives said.

It did seem an odd way to conduct relationships with your children. As if there were things you did not want them to see, or preparations which had to be made before anyone could be admitted to the house.

'What did the sons say about their parents' health?' I asked.

'The mother had cancer about a year ago . . .' He checked his notes. 'Bowel cancer. But she had surgery, got the all-clear about six months ago and she's been fine since.'

'And the father? An alcoholic?'

'Whoa, steady on, Doc, no one's saying that!'

The father was a colonel and, I suspected, his family was his regiment.

'Son just thinks he was showing his age and had got a bit frail; in fact, he described his father as an invalid. Didn't seem to know exactly what was wrong with him.'

'And what was his age?'

'They were both seventy-four.'

This was a surprise. Not only had the Mason-Grants

335

looked older, I would not have expected such frailty, particularly in the well-heeled middle classes, so early. Not without some underlying medical condition. When I was young, seventy-four was certainly old old age, but now . . . maybe my perception has changed as I have aged. Or maybe there really are a lot more active and alert seventy-four-year-olds around than there used to be.

The first of this sad pair to be wheeled in was the wife. There was no evidence of any injuries or attack. But, from her external appearance alone, I suspected that she had died of hypothermia. There was a patchy change in skin colour over some parts of her body – her hips, elbows, knees and hands – to a distinctive red-brown. I have only seen this where hypothermia is present.

'It was bloody cold in there,' the police officers agreed. 'Very cold for May.'

One of them reached for his notebook.

'CSI said his multiple measurements showed that it was never above 13 degrees anywhere in the house at any time during the day.' He paused to turn over a few pages. 'He's, er, asked if you wanted these results as coloured lines on a graph or . . . just a list, Doc?'

He was grinning.

'Oh, coloured lines on a graph, please,' I said. Maybe I shouldn't have banged on quite so much about taking room temperature at that lecture.

'And, Doc, would you like one graph in Fahrenheit and one in Celsius, or –?'

The DCI cut short the banter.

'Look, I can't understand why they didn't just turn on the heating? They weren't poor.'

We shrugged. Perhaps the Mason-Grants were the sort of

couple to turn off the heating at the end of April and on again in October, no matter what the weather in between. I glanced at Mrs Mason-Grant's face. She looked severe. Or perhaps that sharpness around her nose and mouth was just thinness.

The coroner's officer said: 'It doesn't make sense to me. All right, it was chilly, but we're not in the Arctic Circle. You're not telling me this old lady did the shopping, walked back home and then died of cold?'

But the Arctic is not required for hypothermia. It is easy to die of it in your own home if you are old or immobilized: temperatures of 10 degrees Celsius can be lethal, especially if there is a wind or draught or if conditions are damp. I could only assume that Mrs Mason-Grant had returned from the shop and then something had, for an unknown reason, kept her in one spot in the cold hallway.

An internal examination initially revealed a healthy woman. Her respiratory system was fine and her heart was in good shape. Her arteries showed remarkably little atheroma. So little, in fact, for someone her age, that I became suspicious. Cancer seems to mock us sometimes, by apparently doing us the great favour of cleaning up the cardiovascular system, its main rival in the killing game. I wondered if Mrs Mason-Grant's bowel cancer had truly gone away.

I examined her stomach first and found distinctive, diagnostic evidence of hypothermia in the form of tiny black erosions which studded the stomach lining. It looked as though it had been splattered with dark paint. Low temperatures make the blood thicken and it can sludge in the capillaries of many organs. Metabolism in the stomach lining is high and, because it is exposed to large quantities of acids, cells are constantly picked off and then must be replaced.

When the blood supply that fuels this process slows or stops, there are fewer replacement cells and gaps appear in the lining as erosions.

While examining the stomach, I had tried not to look at the nearby liver, although I was constantly aware of it. Vast, colourful. In the corner of my eye, I had the sense of something intrusive, an enormous cuckoo where a dunnock should be. When I had finished with the stomach, I could ignore it no longer. I picked it up.

'What is *that*?' the youngest detective asked.

'Looks like the surface of the moon!' said the coroner's officer, who had seen many a liver.

'I assume that's cirrhosis?' his colleague suggested. 'And that the vodka was for her?'

I shook my head.

'No, I think the vodka was intended to go upstairs to her husband. This liver is full of secondary tumours. Matastases.'

The youngest detective could not take his eyes off such a strange and deformed organ. The tumours varied in size – some were as small as peas and one or two as large as cricket balls. They were dotted throughout, sometimes so close together that their proximity flattened the edges of each tumour as though they were balloons squished together. They were brightly coloured – yellow or red or white or even mottled with all three colours – and the overall effect was quite extraordinary, like something you would find at a grotesque funfair. Its weight was over 3,000 grams. That's more than twice the size of a normal liver.

I checked Mrs Mason-Grant's bowel and found the site of the operation to remove the tumour. It had clearly been successful because there was no evidence of cancer there. She had been given the all-clear but it seemed that, unknown to anyone, it had sneaked out already, into the bloodstream or a lymph node. From there, it had found its way to the liver. But I suspect that Mrs Mason-Grant had guessed this. I soon found out from her doctor that she had recently visited, feeling unwell, and been referred at once for a scan. This had revealed the tumours in her liver . . . but Mrs Mason-Grant had not actually returned to her GP yet for the results. She might have guessed the truth, but she had not been informed of it.

'Can cancer just kill you dead on the spot like that when it spreads to the liver?' asked a detective.

I explained: 'By the time it gets to this stage, the body's internal chemistry will be completely haywire. This cancer is so advanced that it had probably reached a point where the disturbance was just too much.'

'What's your theory then, Doc?' asked the coroner's officer.

'Here's a family that likes to pretend everything's normal – even when it isn't. Mrs Mason-Grant went to the shop every morning, but that morning she must have felt very ill indeed. However, she's of the generation that grits the teeth and follows the usual routines, even though she really didn't want to. I imagine she'd been feeling weak and nauseous for a while, and I expect she was in a lot of abdominal pain. But she probably thought she'd feel better after a walk. Of course, she just felt worse and worse.'

One of the detectives said: 'Yeah, we've talked to the shopkeeper and he wondered if Mrs Mason-Grant was poorly. Because she didn't say anything. She wasn't usually friendly, but at least she was polite.'

'Interestingly, she's not yellow and jaundiced,' I said. 'Quite surprising, in the circumstances, but it happens. Anyway, as

339

she reached the house, she was feeling terrible: we all know how it is when all you want to do is get home and lie down.'

The officers nodded.

'She made it to the front door and put her stick against the wall while she opened it – but never picked it up again. She just closed the door behind her, put down the shopping . . . and then allowed herself to collapse. After that, she couldn't move. She probably didn't want to. In fact, she may well have been unconscious quite quickly. She lay there on the chilly floor, probably in a bit of a draught from the door, and got colder and colder. Until the cold completely engulfed her system. The cold killed her before her liver could – but it probably didn't win by much, and it might have been a dead heat.'

'So how long was she lying there before she died?' asked the youngest detective.

'Probably not much more than an hour,' I said.

'Are you absolutely sure . . .' one of the detectives began. To which the answer is always no, I'm seldom absolutely sure of anything. 'Are you absolutely sure that she didn't get pushed over or attacked by an intruder at the door?'

I said: 'Well, she might have been, but there is no evidence of that. I mean, no bruises, no head injury . . .'

'The sons are making a right fuss . . . they're saying if both parents died at once, then there *must* have been an intruder.'

'And what do they believe has been taken?'

'They're going to the house today to ascertain that.'

I was sure that no one else was involved, but I could understand why the sons thought a double death meant that there must have been some foul play.

The young detective was thinking the same thing.

'Maybe she killed the husband before she died! Before she even went to the shops!'

We all looked at him. Good point.

We agreed that it was time to examine Colonel Mason-Grant.

Her husband was wheeled in as Mrs Mason-Grant was wheeled out.

'Skinny bloke!' the coroner's officer said, staring at the frail body before us.

'Maybe he had cancer too,' a detective suggested.

'And they died of it at the same time?' His colleagues shook their heads. 'Come on!'

I examined him first for cuts or bruises – anything which might indicate that a third person had been in the house, or even, as the detective had suggested, that his wife had attacked him.

He had a couple of old bruises on his chest. There was faint evidence of a bruise on his left temple which, when I looked behind it, revealed an area of bruising that was much bigger and deeper than its outer appearance might have indicated. And, while I was examining the inside of his scalp, I found another major bruise that barely showed on the outside of his head. It was right in the middle at the back.

'Must have been hit on the head!' one of the detectives said excitedly.

'Maybe,' I agreed. 'But more likely he fell backwards on the carpet. He was lying face up.'

Colonel Mason-Grant had none of the skin reddening which is indicative of hypothermia. I examined him very carefully for this, including his hands.

'Look at his nails!' the coroner's officer said. 'Bet he wouldn't show up on parade like that.'

The old soldier's fingernails were long, dirty and distinctively curved. There are some medical words that just seem to

fit the finding and the word for these was onychogryphosis –
which means ram's horn nails.

'I bet he never went out of the house,' someone said. 'Not
looking like that.'

I realized that he might well be right. Colonel Mason-
Grant had presented in life, according to his son, as an
invalid. The reason he could not see his sons without a prior
appointment was that he would have first needed to get up,
get ready . . . and probably get sober for them.

'What was actually wrong with him . . . ?' one of the detectives asked, his tone confused. 'Has anyone told us?'

'Old age,' said another.

'Old age used to be a cause of death, but not now. It's not
a disease,' I reminded him. 'And, so far, I can find absolutely
nothing wrong with him. Respiratory system fine, heart fine,
blood vessels fine, but let's see . . .'

I was examining his stomach now and, sure enough, he
had exactly the same black, splattered-paint lesions as his
wife.

'Oh, that is weird!' said a detective.

'How do we know she didn't give him some kind of poison
to make his stomach spotty and then drink it herself?'
demanded the junior detective, who had obviously been on
one homicide course too many.

'I don't know of any poison that would cause lesions so
typical of hypothermia,' I said.

There was a silence.

'Don't tell me they both died of the same thing,' the coroner's officer said.

I had examined Colonel Mason-Grant's stomach, with the
corner of my eye telling me that all the time there was another
seriously diseased liver waiting for me. I turned to this now.

It was less than a third of the size of his wife's liver. As knobbly as hers but definitely shrunken.

'This is very advanced cirrhosis,' I told them. 'It's showing the battle between scarring and fibrosis and the liver's desperate attempts to regenerate. See the nodules? When I get it under a microscope it's going to look really horrible.'

'So . . . was it hypothermia or was it cirrhosis that killed him?'

'Probably both.'

But two of the detectives were shaking their heads now.

'Same as the wife? Coincidences like that don't happen, Doc,' they said seriously.

'Nothing coincidental about it. The colonel was clearly an alcoholic and his cirrhotic liver would have killed him quite soon. His wife colluded with him to maintain his habit: she probably did as she was told all her married life and now she was told to go shopping. And bring back a bit more than just milk. But one day, she didn't make it up the stairs.'

'So you think that when the tox comes back, it will show he died of alcohol poisoning?'

'No. I think that when the tox comes back it will show he had little or no alcohol in his blood.'

They stared down at Colonel Mason-Grant for a minute, as if he was going to explain to them what had happened.

'Have you ever seen an alcoholic when they can't have a drink?' I asked.

'Yeah. Withdrawal. It's horrible. They start to shake and sometimes they have fits,' the oldest detective said.

'That may have been what happened to the colonel. He heard his wife come home with his alcohol supply, but she was insubordinate and didn't appear. He lay in bed, shouting orders. "Come upstairs immediately!" But she didn't come . . .'

'But there was nothing so much wrong with him, you've

said so!' the young detective exclaimed. 'If the house was cold, there was nothing to stop him turning on the heating. And if he wanted a drink, well, why didn't he go downstairs and get one?'

Before I could reply, his colleague said: 'I reckon his brain was completely addled. She looked after him. She organized everything and ordered a gardener around and told the cleaner what to do, and the colonel didn't show his face to anyone. She did it all. He was helpless.'

'But there was nothing wrong with him except his liver!' repeated the junior.

'With this degree of cirrhosis, there was certainly something wrong with him. He might have had psychosis caused by alcohol, for all we know,' I said.

'He was a drunk, and they were ashamed,' said the coroner's officer. 'They couldn't even admit it to their own sons. Had to get him out of the bedroom, dress him, clean his fingernails and prop him up in a chair before the lads could come home to visit their parents.'

I said: 'When his wife didn't come, maybe he did try to go downstairs. I doubt he was curious or worried about her so much as keen to get the vodka. But he didn't make it past the bed. He collapsed. He may have had a fit; anyway, he certainly bumped his head. And probably lay there for a long time without food or drink. In the cold. Until he died.'

'So . . . they both collapsed because of their livers. And died because of the cold,' the senior detective said slowly.

'Well, I'm open to any other scenario you can think of that fits the medical facts.'

There was a little more discussion of intruders, but it was half-hearted and I could see that the officers were beginning to accept my version of events.

'Interesting pair of livers they had in that house,' I said as we took off our scrubs.

The next morning, the investigating officer phoned me and asked me if I would meet with the three sons. They still believed there must have been an intruder – although they had to admit that nothing seemed to be missing from the house.

We met in my office at the hospital. The three sons were very different. The eldest worked in the City, wore a suit, spoke seriously in a low voice and conducted himself with great restraint, in the manner, I suspected, of his father. The middle son wore torn jeans and had many tattoos and pier-cings. It was easy to imagine some angry confrontations with his parents, evidently people who were devoted to keeping up appearances. The youngest was relaxed and friendly: he said he worked for a film company and he cried during our interview, the only son who felt able to show an emotional response to their parents' deaths. It was evident that none of them had chosen to follow their father into the army. I won-dered if that had been a disappointment to their parents, and if they had shown that disappointment.

The three of them were very different but they were united in their insistence that two deaths could only have occurred at the same time as a result of third-party intrusion. I gently pointed out that Colonel and Mrs Mason-Grant had not, in fact, died at the same time. Their father had died many hours after their mother. But since neither body had shown even the smallest sign of decomposition and there had been some rigor mortis still present in just the legs of both of the deceased, I was sure they had both died on Tuesday, or, given the cold, possibly Monday.

This prompted considerable angst in the youngest son.

Until now, he had assumed that his parents had died over the weekend. Now he realized that, if he had only dared to visit the house on Monday, he might have arrived in time to save them. Of course, his parents had instilled in him the belief that he must not do so. Their deaths, as so often, were a product of their lives and personalities. But that did not help the youngest son. His misery was acute. The middle brother was quick to comfort him; the eldest looked embarrassed.

'There was nothing you could have done,' I said. How often I have used those words to reassure heartbroken relatives who are hounded by a sense of guilt. 'Your mother's liver cancer was at a very advanced stage indeed.'

'Why didn't she say?' the youngest son howled.

'Because,' the middle son told him, 'she never said anything. She'd only been *his* mouthpiece for fifty years.'

'There seems to have been a lot of stiff upper lip in your family,' I suggested. 'And to be fair, she didn't know. She'd only just had a scan . . .'

'She didn't tell us!'

'. . . and had not yet been given the results. But that would not have been pleasant news to receive. Her GP would have told her that there was no treatment at this stage and that death was very close.'

'Did she guess?'

'Probably. She must have felt extremely ill. It's astonishing she made it to the shop and back. As for your father . . . well . . . I assume you know that he was an alcoholic.'

They did not respond but, from their faces, it was clear that the whole family knew. Although everyone pretended not to. They had acquiesced to the façade of old-age frailty that their father presented when they visited because each brother, independently, must have reached the conclusion

346

that this was the least painful way of dealing with a painful situation.

'He was the boss, she carried out his orders,' said the middle son, an edge of anger in his voice. 'Nothing was going to change that.'

'We never should have left her to cope with him alone!' the youngest son said.

'She insisted,' the eldest son reminded him. 'It was her choice.'

'I'm trying to tell you,' I said, 'that both your parents were very ill. Your father's cirrhotic liver really could not have been functioning properly and he almost certainly only had a short time to live. Your mother's liver cancer was inoperable and took its natural course. If you had arrived earlier in the week, you might have saved them from hypothermia – which, incidentally, is probably not a bad or painful way to die – only for them to be killed by their livers very soon afterwards.'

The youngest son sniffed. I wanted to remind him of our life's great and inevitable cycle and how an important part of it is this: our parents die. Their death is a time for grief but also retrospection and a recognition that the cycle turns constantly and that, in time, we, too, must age and die.

But soon he was in floods of tears, the middle brother was hugging him and the eldest was looking extremely awkward. Perhaps now was not the moment to talk about life's great cycle.

Double deaths are rare, but not as rare as you might think. They most frequently arise when older people have reached a state of high dependency. When the stronger of the two collapses unexpectedly, the weaker is left to fend for him or herself. Sometimes a double death occurs when the weaker partner – who is often up in the bedroom – rushes downstairs at an unaccustomed pace to investigate the silence of the stronger partner – and breaks their neck. Double deaths like these are a symptom of dependency, and dependency is a symptom of something unwelcome but inevitable – the fact that, as time passes, senescence progresses.

I am already trying to recognize and prepare myself for the limitations that old old age will bring to my life one day. To develop an interest for the time when my knees prevent me from walking far and when, perish the thought, cognitive decline means that I cannot be trusted at the controls of a small plane.

I am lucky that there is something I love to do which is possible when sitting down in a warm environment. I have started to restore old clocks. I have repaired a few beauties already and I am studying to become a technician in horology. It gives me great pleasure to enter this new world and to learn about it. Horology will keep me productively entertained and engaged when physical frailty contracts my world. Until, of course, the arthritis in my hands stops me.

19

Here are three cases in which all of the deceased are old, and I do not mean young old. I chose them almost at random from dozens – no, hundreds – of similar cases. You will find the medicine in them quite straightforward. Morally and legally – which, of course, are not always the same thing – they are much more complex.

Case one is eighty-one-year-old Godfrey Oliver. He and his wife lived near the sea and were thinking about going to bed one evening when there was a knock at the door. Mrs Oliver answered it, and an intruder stormed into the house. He was carrying a kitchen knife. Shouting loudly, he threatened Mrs Oliver and then proceeded to the living room, where he found Mr Oliver sitting on the sofa and, with no apparent motive, began to attack him with fists and knife. That the intruder, who was known to the Olivers only as a distant neighbour, was mentally ill or very drunk is not in doubt: in fact, he was very drunk.

The suddenness, volume and ferocity of such an attack would be terrifying for anyone, but Mrs Oliver had the presence of mind to call the police, at which point the intruder stumbled off into the night.

The police and ambulance arrived to find Godfrey Oliver with cuts and bruises and his wife with a minor stab wound to her pelvis. Of course, both were very shocked.

All their injuries could have been serious, but the local hospital quickly established that none was. They did recognize, however, how destabilizing such an event can be in the lives of the very old. Mrs Oliver's history is not recorded, but her husband was admitted and treated for his injuries and then sent to another, larger, nearby hospital which had an observation ward. He was clearly both distressed and unwell and he remained under the care and observation of the hospital for almost a month before his condition deteriorated and he died.

The police were keen to prosecute the intruder not just for assault, but now also for murder. You might think that manslaughter would be more appropriate: the intruder caused no great physical harm to Mr Oliver and he had no way of knowing that Mr Oliver was greatly weakened by lung cancer. But that is not a defence in law. According to the law, an assailant 'must take his victim as he finds them', which means that beating up someone who subsequently dies is considered to be murder, whatever the perpetrator knew or did not know about the victim's ill health.

At post-mortem, the first thing I noticed about Godfrey Oliver was his extreme thinness. He was not short, but he weighed only 32 kilos, not far from the average weight of a ten-year-old. On external examination, I did not find physical evidence of the attack: his injuries had evidently healed. But, internally, I found that he had suffered a small brain haemorrhage which was not yet fully resolved.

His heart was not in bad shape for his age and his coronary arteries were only moderately blocked. But in the mighty aorta there was a distinct build-up of plaque in just one area. Here the arterial wall was ballooning on to the abdomen. It was an aneurysm just waiting to rupture.

However, the cradle of his ill health was not this point of extreme vulnerability but his lungs. First, there was a tumour.

This had reached the size of six centimetres, although it was so poorly delineated that it was hard to know where the tumour stopped and lung tissue began. I have already described the crab-like appearance of tumours, and Mr Oliver's was very crabby, with claws stretching in all directions. Hard, menacing, its colour white and yellow variegated, it was flecked with red and black. Cells had died and were decomposing at its centre already because it was growing so fast that its developing blood supply could not keep pace. And, where degeneration was taking place, here the tumour was a soft, soggy mass.

Mr Oliver had been diagnosed a few months earlier and, although it had been agreed that full, curative treatment was not an option, he had been offered some radiotherapy to extend his life. He had been due to start this in the month that he died.

The tumour was bad enough, his arterial disease also, but Mr Oliver in addition had very serious emphysema. It might have resulted from his industrial occupation, although it is more likely that the main cause was his heavy smoking. Emphysema makes the lungs at first glance look very holey indeed. Healthy lungs are like firm, pink bath sponges: this is true of children, but even some elderly people, non-smokers from a non-polluted rural environment, do manage to maintain that pink-bath-sponge health all their lives.

Where there is emphysema, the sponge becomes increasingly full of holes of all sizes – some may be as large as cricket balls. I can pick the edge of emphysematous lungs up with my forceps and look straight through them and easily imagine that I am looking through a dirty dishcloth.

In death, the emphysematous lungs are sad, deflated things, flat as a collapsed soufflé. I can simulate life simply by pushing formalin into them. I did this and, hey presto, now the holes were blown out and fixed, as if Mr Oliver had just taken a deep breath and was holding it.

Once the two-dimensional holes were three-dimensional bubbles, it was obvious how the tissue between the tiny air sacs, the alveoli, had broken down and how the air sacs had joined and joined again to make larger and larger bubbles. In fact, Mr Oliver's lungs were essentially just bubbles – pea size, golf-ball size and, yes, cricket balls too. How he must have struggled for breath, because, as these huge parodies of air sacs increase, the total surface area decreases, until they can offer no useful gas exchange.

The best way to really examine lungs is to slice them into thin slivers. And now here was something wonderful. I experienced the same pleasure as I do on glimpsing an apple tree hanging with gorgeous red fruit growing by a rubbish tip. No matter how ugly tumours, chronic obstructive pulmonary disease or emphysematous lungs sound, they are an example of the way nature chooses the most hideous places to reveal her great beauty.

In cross-section, Mr Oliver's lungs were made of lace. The many bubbles, of different diameters and uneven shape, created fine lines of extraordinary and eccentric loveliness. The lacemaker was mad, drunk perhaps, but outstandingly talented. And here, to one side of the slice, was the shimmering white, yellow, red and black of the tumour, its tentacles stretching through the fine filigree like elegantly gloved fingers.

Mr Oliver can have had no idea of the beauty of his lungs and he had lost consciousness by the time that beauty killed him. Although, precisely, it was neither the cancer nor the emphysema that had ended his life. No, the true killer is known as Old Folks' Friend. I knew as soon as I handled his lungs, without even putting them under a microscope, that he had contracted bronchopneumonia in hospital. It was like feeling dried peas scattered through both lungs. Grains the size of sugar join together to become bigger until they reach pea size – they do not get as large as golf or cricket balls – and these are the evidence, the discarded cannonballs left on the battlefield, of Mr Oliver's white cells magnificently fighting to defend him against bacterial infection. But, of course, they eventually did lose the battle.

Was his pneumonia caused because he was immobilized for so long? He was, after all, confined to a hospital bed as a direct result of the assault. Or was it caused, as it certainly can be, by his underlying lung cancer?

In other words, how direct is the link between the sudden arrival of a drunken, knife-wielding intruder into the Olivers' home and the death of Godfrey Oliver almost one month later? Would he have died when he did without such an attack?

You might think the answer to that question is no. You might argue that, despite his ill health, Mr Oliver may have had months – even, with the proposed radiotherapy and good luck, a whole year – left to live, had the attack not happened.

If the police argued that to the Crown Prosecution Service, they were disappointed. The CPS decided that neither a charge of murder, nor even of manslaughter, would be successful in court. The intruder did face less serious assault charges, but he was never prosecuted for the death of Godfrey Oliver.

Case 2 is Emanuel Adebyo. After changing a flat tyre on his car on a hot day he approached his house tired and dishevelled. He was seventy-nine years old. I do not have any record of the reason why his next-door neighbours decided to pick a fight with him at this time, but police notes indicate that Mr Adebyo was undoubtedly an innocent party in the argument.

The verbal abuse he received grew serious. And then one of the aggressive neighbours threw a punch, quite a nasty one. Mr Adebyo staggered but held on to the fence and did not fall. He was a devout Christian and was able to look at his attackers and tell them, quietly, that he forgave them. But within a minute he had collapsed.

During the altercation, his wife, scared to leave the house, had called the police. Therefore, they were on the spot very soon after her husband hit the ground: in fact, when Mrs Adebyo dared to come out of the door, she found the police attempting resuscitation.

An ambulance took the patient straight to hospital, where a crash team was waiting. They had already seen his notes and learned that he had high blood pressure and had been treated for heart arrhythmia two years before.

The crash team resuscitated him and stabilized his cardio-vascular system, but he remained deeply unconscious. Consciousness is measured using the Glasgow Coma Scale, which assesses eye opening, verbal response and motor response. The maximum possible score is fifteen and the minimum is three. Mr Adebyo scored three.

The crash team were worried about a possible head injury, either as a result of the punch or from hitting his head as he fell. However, a CT scan showed no fractures or haemorrhage inside the skull. His GCS remained at three. His pupils were fixed and dilated and did not react to light. There was no response to voice. And he showed no motor responses: he could not breathe when disconnected from a ventilator.

The following day, consultant neurologists and a neuro-surgeon clustered around his bed. They reviewed the situation, the CT scans and his current clinical condition and declared the situation hopeless. And they ordered brain-stem tests to see if there was any response. These tests are per-formed by two separate and independent doctors, the second test some hours after the first, to prevent errors – and collusion.

The tests confirmed that Mr Adebyo was brain dead and that there was no chance of recovery. The changes on the CT showed widespread damage and swelling throughout the whole brain, and they believed this had been caused not by the blow itself, or even by the fall. They felt it resulted from that period, before the police and paramedics started to resuscitate him, when Mr Adebyo was in cardiac arrest and his brain was starved of oxygen.

His life could only be prolonged artificially. Mr Adebyo's family, who were also devout Christians, were, like so many in this situation, hoping for a miracle. But it was pointed out to them that prolonging life mechanically would not change matters and was not really in anyone's interests. The family then faced an exceptionally hard decision. To them, it simply appeared that he was asleep – apart from the tubes and the ventilator.

Almost exactly five days after the blow had been struck, Mr Adebyo's family, helped by the hospital chaplain and their own pastor, were able to accept that the brain damage was irreversible. They were present at Mr Adebyo's death when medical support was withdrawn. And, at that moment, the criminal charges against the neighbours turned from attempted murder into murder.

I carried out the first post-mortem.

There was clear evidence of the punch to the victim's face in the faint external bruise on his left cheek. Internally, this bruise was deep and prominent, measuring about seven centimetres square. There were healing abrasions on the back of his head and on the left side of his back. And beneath all these abrasions were deep bruises which were typical of a fall on to the back.

Internally, the brain's outer, mountainous landscape had become flattened, as if a glacier had passed over it. This is exactly what you would expect to find in someone whose body has been kept alive when the brain has been starved of oxygen. However, I found no evidence of a haemorrhage on the surface of the brain or deep within it.

Apart from this, Mr Adebyo had been a healthy seventy-nine-year-old in all respects except one. That coronary artery, the left anterior descending, the one of the three coronary arteries most prone to blocking: at one point, I found Mr Adebyo's was 90 per cent obstructed by atheroma. And on top of the blockage was a blood clot. A thrombosis. Here was a classic coronary artery thrombosis over classic coronary artery atheroma. That part of the heart muscle supplied by the artery must suddenly have been deprived of oxygen when the blood clot formed.

One other finding was recent rib fractures. But these were not sinister: in fact, broken ribs are entirely to be expected when the police or paramedics desperately try to save a life.

I agreed with the neurologists that the damage to the brain had been caused not by the blow or the fall but by lack of oxygen during the time when Mr Adebyo's heart had stopped beating. He might, in a technical sense, have been killed ultimately by brain damage – but the blockage in the coronary artery had caused a myocardial infarction, a heart attack, which stopped his heart from beating. This was the first link in the chain of events leading to his death.

So, the question then was not what had happened but when had it happened. The myocardial infarction could be dated at pretty much exactly five days before his ultimate death – in other words, to the day of the attack.

This indication of a heart attack at – or about – the time of the argument meant that the CPS were now happy to proceed with murder charges. As I'd performed the first examination on Mr Adebyo and advised the police, I found myself in court as an expert witness for the prosecution. I guessed there would be some robust cross-examination and I planned to present my stance on the case early, during my initial questioning by the prosecution barrister. English law may say that you must take your victims as you find them, but there are defence barristers who still try, and occasionally manage, to drive a cart and horses through this concept. In my experience of such prosecutions, the longer between collapse and death, the lower the chance of success. And in this case, there had been five days, so I could expect a challenge.

Of course, the defence, after reading my post-mortem report, was keen to argue that the neighbours' action had contributed almost nothing to Mr Adebyo's death: with a coronary artery blockage like that, they argued, he was already a death waiting to happen.

Yes, I agreed under cross-examination, Mr Adebyo could have died at any time from his severe heart disease. But I was quick to add that he, equally, could have lived for years. I had examined the bodies of people who died of other causes and who were much older than Mr Adebyo, and their degree of atheroma had been just as bad or even worse.

I had earlier explained, at the request of the prosecution

barrister, how stress causes us to release adrenaline. This hormone reduces the blood supply to all non-essential organs in the body to maximize the blood flow, and therefore oxygen, to the skeletal muscles, the brain and to the heart – in case we need to run or fight for our lives. And the heart is badly in need of oxygen because, thanks to the adrenaline, it is beating much faster. We are all familiar with that loud, hard thumping in the chest when we experience fear.

If the heart's blood supply is restricted by a blockage when the heart is beating so hard, parts of the heart muscle may become deprived of oxygen. The heart may well now beat in a dangerously irregular way. As in Mr Adebyo's case, the arrhythmia can cause collapse – which may, of course, result in an impact to the head. If death is immediate, no obvious damage to the heart muscle will be seen. But Mr Adebyo actually 'lived' for five days in ICU and so the body's repair processes in his damaged heart muscle continued for that period.

The defence wanted to know which Mr Adebyo had found more stressful: the verbal abuse he was subjected to or the punch in the face. I said that verbal abuse alone could have raised adrenaline to a dangerous level but that the pain of the blow would also have released dangerous amounts of adrenaline: that is one result of pain.

What about the hot weather? the barrister persisted. What about the flat tyre? Wasn't that all stressful? As nothing, I insisted, compared to the stress of abuse and a punch.

So, why had the victim not collapsed immediately? Why did he have enough time to converse with his attackers before falling to the ground, if adrenaline had increased his heart rate so much? I said that the release of adrenaline would have continued even when the stressor events had stopped.

And, for a long time, it would certainly have continued to cause the major cardiovascular changes it is designed for. I pointed out that after a shock, even after non-traumatic stress, the raised pulse, the pounding of the heart and the sensation of fear may continue for many minutes.

But counsel was a dog with a bone. He creased his face into one of those cartoon expressions of disbelief which I suppose they teach them in law school. *Surely*, he said, *surely*, I should be able to distinguish between the stress caused by the argument and the stress caused by the punch?

This was ridiculous, but the jousting went on for some time. Simply declining to answer a question put to you in court is not an option for an expert witness. No matter how stupid the question. I opted for the multiple negative approach.

'I am not able to say with certainty that, if the blow had not been struck, collapse could not have occurred.'

The barrister could hardly hide his smile.

I added that *surely* we needed to consider the incident as a whole because the two events were so related in time that they *surely* could not be separated.

But I think the barrister was too busy licking his lips to notice.

In language that was unusually strong for me, I stated: 'However, I would also say that the proposition that death was inevitable following the verbal abuse alone, and that the blows can therefore be excluded, is totally erroneous. Both must be relevant.'

By now the barrister was waving an old medical textbook from some dusty library. He had been reading about silent infarcts and knew it was possible to have a heart attack and not even notice . . . not for a while, anyway. I had timed Mr Adebyo's heart attack to the day of the incident, but how could I know precisely that it had not happened before the argument had even started, when he was changing the flat tyre in the merciless glare of the high summer sun (like many barristers, he was a novelist *manqué*)? Unless, of course . . . (here he again adopted a face of cartoon cunning) I was clever enough to time the heart attack to the very minute it had happened.

I said: 'The size of the area damaged in the heart was so great that it is highly unlikely it would not have been painful. And therefore hardly silent.'

The barrister opened his mouth to speak, but I was quick.

'And, almost certainly, Mr Adebyo would have become breathless as his heart stopped working efficiently. I really do not think such an event could have gone unnoticed by him.'

There was a long pause before the barrister started again. Tirelessly. I believe it is important to recognize and acknowledge, with humility, the full range of life's possibilities. This philosophy has got me into a lot of hot water in court. There are times when it has seemed to me that the courtroom winners are the bombastic, the stubborn and the insistent. And I'm not one of them.

In response to the barrister's continued insistence that Mr Adebyo might have had a silent infarct while changing the tyre, I finally said: 'I cannot exclude absolutely the possibility that there had been a random spontaneous area of heart muscle damage prior to the altercation. But there was no evidence of such damage microscopically and the area of muscle damaged is entirely consistent with a single, large event.'

During his summing up, defence counsel was looking very pleased with himself. The judge reminded the jury that they must not find the defendants guilty if they had any doubt at all that the neighbours were responsible for the death of Mr Adebyo. The jury had doubt. They found the neighbours not guilty.

I was cross with myself when the case was over because I felt I had risen to goading by counsel. Perhaps I hadn't explained the complexities of the pathology well enough to the jury, although I knew that a jury made entirely of doctors who understood the medical details would have had a hard enough time reaching a decision. I felt sorry for Mrs Adebyo, though, when the case ended. How terrible it must have been for her to continue to live next door to her neighbours.

Case three started with an incident in a supermarket car park. Ernest Colebrook, aged seventy-eight, lived nearby, had finished his shopping and was now on his way home. The shortest route took him through the car park. And Ernest would certainly have taken the shortest route: he was quite doddery, by all accounts.

At the same time, Richard White, age twenty-six, finished his shopping. He had heard the siren call of alcohol while at a friend's house, borrowed a car and rushed off for a bottle of rum and a packet of cigarettes. He had drawn attention to himself in the supermarket for his rudeness to staff. Now he was reversing rapidly from his space without taking the trouble to look behind him. He had almost completed the arc of the turn when he hit Ernest Colebrook.

Afterwards, he said he was unaware of this. He sped out of the car park, the entire incident having been recorded on CCTV.

Passers-by rushed to Ernest's aid. An ambulance was called, and so were the police.

Happily, it turned out that Ernest's injuries, though painful and a great inconvenience, were not life-threatening. His right tibia, which runs from the knee down to the ankle and is otherwise called the shin bone, was fractured just below the knee – a classic 'bumper bar' injury. There was an operation to repair the fracture, after which Ernest was not to leave the hospital for some days. When he did leave, of course he wore a plaster cast, which greatly restricted his mobility. Immobility is one of the main causes of deep vein thrombosis.

Veins don't have a pump of their own to get blood back to the heart. They rely on the movements of the body, that is, muscle contractions, which drive the blood up through a series of flap valves designed to prevent back flow. If the muscles don't move for some time, the veins aren't squeezed and the blood may pool in the vein. Pooled, static blood has a tendency to form a clot.

There are many risk factors for DVT, or VTE, venous thromboembolism, as it is sometimes now called. In many cases, immobility is the most significant trigger; a few people have a genetic predisposition to clot, but it really can be precipitated by almost anything – from an infection like Covid-19 to cancer to obesity. The first sign, if there is any sign at all, is a swollen, red leg.

Blood clots are dangerous in any vessel anywhere in the body. In the veins, the clots can break away from the wall and travel up the increasingly large vessels to the heart, where they pass through the right ventricle. On the next leg of their journey, towards the lungs, the vessels get progressively smaller. Sooner or later, the clot will be the same size as the vessel. At which point it gets stuck, blocking the flow of blood to the lungs. This is a pulmonary embolism, and it can be life-threatening. That a pulmonary embolism follows a deep venous thrombosis is not quite so certain as night following day, but anyone hearing the words 'deep venous thrombosis' must recognize the strong possibility of that consequence.

For Ernest Colebrook, night did follow day. As he sat at home, immobilized by the plaster on his leg, his carers should, perhaps, have been more alert to the likelihood of finding thrombosis here. Maybe his left leg, under the plaster, was in fact red and swollen anyway, but I found later that he had deep vein thrombosis in the other leg, too. And why should someone have been checking? Because he had already demonstrated a tendency to develop clots in his leg veins.

Five years earlier, he had experienced a series of small pulmonary emboli. He was prescribed a blood thinner, an anti-coagulant, to prevent repetition of the problem. For five years, it had worked. But not now. He had not one but two DVTs which had become detached and embedded in his lungs. The police did not at all like Richard White, who had been driving without insurance, and they were keen to head their list of charges with causing death by dangerous driving. They were disappointed to find that their chance of a successful prosecution was diminished rather than increased by alcohol, since there was so much of it involved in the incident: Richard White had a bottle of rum in the car and his breath test was positive, but his blood test showed that he was very slightly lower than the English ethanol limit of 80 mg/100 ml. In addition, Mr Colebrook's shopping bags turned out to be full of very strong beer and some cheap wine. No one had tested his blood alcohol level when he arrived in hospital, but a nurse noted that his breath might have smelled of alcohol.

The defence would certainly make good use of her assessment and the contents of his shopping bag to suggest that

Ernest Colebrook had drunkenly wandered behind the reversing car. The defence would also make hay with my post-mortem comments about Ernest Colebrook's liver. It was greatly enlarged and showed the chronic fatty change associated with alcohol use. In addition, his body's main artery, the aorta, carried so much atheroma that in one place it was bulging dangerously. Here, yet again, was a rupture waiting to happen. The heart was greatly enlarged as a result of long-term high blood pressure and, indeed, there was also evidence of the scars from old heart attacks, although nothing recent.

Ernest Colebrook died thirteen days after the car-park incident. To me, the chain of events was as clear as the ancient nursery rhyme in which, for want of a nail, the kingdom is ultimately lost.

As a direct result of Richard White's car hitting him, Mr Colebrook's leg was broken. As a direct result of this broken leg, he was immobilized. As a direct result of immobilization, he developed deep venous thrombosis (although he admittedly had a history of thrombosis). As a direct result of venous thrombosis, he suffered from pulmonary emboli. And as a direct result of these pulmonary emboli, he died. *Quod erat demonstrandum.*

I received a letter from the Crown Prosecution Service, whose job it is to decide if the state is likely to win a case or if pressing charges would just be wasting taxpayers' money on a lost cause.

The CPS lawyer had no time at all for phrases like 'taking your victim as you find them'. She pointed out that, according to case precedents, the original incident must be a 'substantial cause of death'. She didn't think anyone could call a broken leg a substantial cause of a death when that death had occurred thirteen days later due to emboli.

I sighed. Evidently my post-mortem report was not clear enough because she did not understand the direct line of causation from a broken leg through DVT to a pulmonary embolism. At the end of the letter, she reminded me that all prosecutions must be in the public interest.

Personally, I felt that charging Richard White might well be in the public interest, but I stuck to things medical when I phoned her to explain my comments.

'But how much is the broken leg really directly responsible for Mr Colebrook's death?' she repeated.

I said that I believed that the car hitting the leg was at least 80 per cent responsible. I was excluding 20 per cent only because I could not be completely sure of the part played by Ernest's earlier DVT. Would he be alive today if he had not been hit by a car? Almost certainly. I said I hoped that she would consider 80 per cent substantial enough.

'Just a minute. You said: *almost* certainly? You're only *almost* certain he would be alive?'

I said: 'Well, he did have bad heart disease. But who can ever be wholly certain of anything? I can't be absolutely a hundred per cent sure that I'll get home safely tonight, can I?'

But, by now, I had guessed the outcome. And, sure enough, the police rang me soon afterwards in great disappointment to say that the CPS had told them that they would prosecute Richard White for driving without insurance but not for the death of Ernest Colebrook.

In each of these three cases, dying seems a response which is disproportionate, or separate from, the physical damage inflicted by the alleged perpetrator. But dying with little provocation is something the very old are apt to do. Does that make the perpetrators any less guilty?

Apparently so, because in not one of these three cases was

anyone who might have caused the death charged or held in any way responsible for it, although, in each case, had the initial incident not occurred, the victim would *almost* certainly have lived on.

While the same rules apply to anyone, the fact is that in this sort of case the victim is usually old. Why are perpetrators so seldom held to account for the death of old folk? Is it because we consider the lives of the elderly expendable? Or simply because, by the time humans reach old age, there are so many systems malfunctioning that death sits at the awkward and confusing interface of a perpetrator's action and a victim's weakness?

20

The other day I was fixing a leak under the kitchen sink. I had to lie down to look up at the pipes. It had taken a little while and several ungainly manoeuvres to get down there and, once on the floor, I knew I had made a very bad mistake. Job done, but when I tried to stand up again I could do so only by rolling over on to my knees, crouching backwards and then moving one leg forward at a time. With my hands assisting.

Then last night I tried to open a jar. My fingers – the ones with the Heberden's nodes which indicated early arthritic changes twenty years ago – refused to grip the lid tightly enough. Sweating and swearing did not help. Eventually, by wedging the lid of the jar between the door and its frame, I managed to open it. I had found, once again, that I could issue a command to my body which it was unable to carry out.

So, I thought, here it comes. Old old age.

In the last two years, it isn't just arthritis that has worsened. I have also been treated for prostate cancer. This is a very common cancer. When I was training to be a pathologist, the rule of thumb was that, if you looked hard enough, you could find a focus of cancerous cells in the prostate of at least 80 per cent of males over the age of eighty. But, while clearly malignant, most would be so innocuous that they would seldom be the cause of death. However, there are certainly more aggressive forms: the exact course of the disease may well be determined by genes.

My father's prostate cancer was diagnosed in his sixties

and he died as a result of it in his eighties. My brother, happily still well, also had prostate cancer in his sixties. Naturally, I deluded myself that I would be the one male of the family not to have it. So I dodged my Prostate-Specific Antigen test. Then, one day, I developed an infection which was extremely painful, particularly on urination. I went to see my GP. I thought the antibiotics he gave me would clear it up in a few days. They didn't.

'Odd,' said the GP. 'There weren't any bugs in your wee. So we'll repeat that test. Leave a sample before you go.'

The GP gave me a course of different antibiotics. I felt awful. I developed a fever and just wanted to curl up in bed and be semi-conscious. It took a third visit and the antibiotic equivalent of Domestos before the infection, prostatitis, began to budge. As soon as I was well, I was keen to forget the whole incident.

But the difficulty in eradicating the infection should have been a red flag. My prostate might as well have held up a large sign saying: check me for cancer! The hospital wanted to do just that, but I preferred not to read the sign. I just wanted to get on with life and I really didn't have time for a complication like cancer when I felt fine.

Of course, I finally had a Prostate-Specific Antigen test and the result was very high. That's normal after a fierce infection. The prostate is the walnut-sized gland just below the bladder which creates the seminal fluid necessary for ejaculation. As well as sperm, urine passes through it on the way out. It is hormone-driven, the hormone being of course testosterone, and, like most glands, this means cell regeneration occurs at a brisk rate. The higher the rate of cell division, the wider the door is open to mistakes. And cancer is one big mistake.

Unfortunately, the high PSA didn't go down. By now, my

doctor was extremely suspicious. You might think that I would have delighted in his concern, but I was very slow indeed to agree to an MRI scan.

It showed that, yes, things did not look right with my prostate.

I thought: well, obviously, that's just a bit of scarring from the infection.

It was all very annoying. But, finally, I had to agree to a biopsy.

When I was told that I did have cancer, I realized how I had been living in a fool's paradise. I hoped I didn't have cancer. I didn't want to have cancer. Therefore, I wouldn't have cancer. And even when everything pointed to it, from the infection onwards, I had continued to row down the river called denial.

By this time, I scored annoyingly high on the Gleason grading system, which is an assessment for the aggression of prostate cancer. Under a microscope, the cancer's various levels of intensity (these can vary even in one tumour) are qualified and quantified. The scale was initially from one to ten, but it is now refined and reduced to a more practically useful scale of six to nine. My score was seven.

A Gleason seven score equates to a grade-two cancer. This is quite mild and treatable, but grade one would have been better and, if not for my obstinance, my idiotic hope and denial, I probably would have been a grade one.

I was given a choice between radiotherapy and surgery. You mean, someone in scrubs and mask would be standing over me with a scalpel the way I stand over the deceased at post-mortem? No, thanks. I chose radiotherapy. First a day operation under anaesthetic where computer-controlled radioactive needles delivered a knockout blow to my prostate.

Followed by a quick, daily dose of radiotherapy for two weeks from a sophisticated X-ray machine. It became almost a social event with the team at the hospital. That was two years ago, and now I feel fit and healthy and grateful that the NHS was more persistent in pursuit of my health than I was.

So, it's all over then, I thought, when I was given the all-clear again at my latest review. Until . . . a few months ago I found myself looking at blood on the loo paper and swearing. Oh-oh. Some unwanted side effect of radiotherapy? This time, I went straight into action.

The bleeding was not a complication of the radiotherapy but a whole separate problem. In my bowel. I submitted, gracefully, to the indignity of a colonoscopy. A benign polyp was found and, since any cell overgrowth can rapidly turn nasty, it was removed. I was able to watch the entire process, fascinated, on a screen. When the surgeon marked the inside of my bowel with a small tattoo, I felt quite joyful. Another one of life's little mysteries solved. I had wondered for years why I sometimes found these small blue marks in people's bowels. How on earth did they get there? Now I knew. Surgeons mark the point of removal in case any further polyps develop.

I would rather not admit it but, since reaching my mid-sixties, I have to recognize that health issues have begun to stack up.

My life's work witnessing man's inhumanity to man finally did culminate in a snapping of fault lines, a process I have documented elsewhere. After the earthquake, when I had been diagnosed with post-traumatic stress disorder, I seriously contemplated suicide. I have often stood over the body of someone who died this way, wondering how they could cause such suffering to their loved ones. Now at last I understood that so little beyond their own pain exists for the suicidal that they may not be aware of their loved ones at all. When I contemplated killing myself in front of a train, it had to be gently pointed out to me that this would cause the train driver suffering for the rest of their life. It simply had not occurred to me, although I have examined plenty of people who died this way and I know how hideous the consequences are for the body and – of course – the train driver. That is the closed world of suicide and I was lucky to receive enough help to bring me back to this other, happier world.

Then there was that low-grade and easily treatable cancer. The swiftly despatched bowel polyp. My idiotic fall from a ladder and resulting concussion. Worsening arthritis. My ludicrous flirtation with alcohol. And, most recently, cysts on my liver requiring investigation. I recite this list with regret, aware that, after six decades in which I barely visited my GP, there is an inevitability with age of compounding health worries. A series of inconveniences. A roadmap of senescence. Harbingers for the future. If anyone had told me ten years ago that I would accumulate such a series of small misadventures, I would not have believed them. The accumulation is entirely normal at this age. But none of us thinks it will happen to us.

We fool ourselves if we think we can cheat ageing. There are celebrities who work out for hours in an attempt to maintain their youth or who pay immense sums for plastic surgery, but the fact is that we instinctively know their age bracket at one glance, because our age is written on us, whatever we do to erase the evidence. We lose the elasticity in our skin and it wrinkles, our hands show pigment changes, we certainly lose our body hair and probably some of the hair on our heads, too, we often put on weight and, even if we don't, fat shifts to different places in our bodies so that our outline is different, our muscles look different and we move differently.

371

The inside of the body, however, at first glance seems similar to our much younger body. And, if there are changes, many of them are optional. That bulging arterial wall, threatening to break with the quantity of plaque and atheroma blocking the vessel: we could have eaten a better diet, only we didn't. That fatty liver: we could have drunk less, only we didn't. Those grey, holey lungs: we could have given up smoking, only we didn't. Of course, much of this is genetic. But not all of it. Now we are very old, our life's story, our habits, our behaviours, our likes and dislikes, they are here inside us, telling our story and foretelling how we will die.

I looked at the body of Mrs Doreen Lowe, aged eighty-six, and tried to read her story. Her womb told me that she had given birth to at least two children; her ovaries told me that this had been long ago. Her missing spleen, the ghost of a break in her left ribs and the slightest blush of a resolved brain haemorrhage told me that an accident, I wondered if it might have been a road traffic accident, had befallen her in the past, probably in midlife. Her dentition and cardiovascular system said that she had enjoyed her food, especially buttery, sweet food like cakes and pastries. Her liver confirmed that she drank only a little. Her pink lungs boasted that she had never smoked or lived in a dirty, polluted city like London. Her arthritis in the hip said that she had been partially immobilized in her later years and it had perhaps contributed to her weight gain: much of this weight she carried around her abdomen.

The exterior of her body, when she was first wheeled in, had shown me a little more. Evidently, she had led a comfortable and well-ordered life. She kept her fingernails clean and filed, her neat grey hair spoke of regular visits to the salon, her clothes were in good order. She had cloudy eyes and a distinctive arcus senilis – the white ring which shows sometimes around the iris of the elderly. It is composed of, among other things, cholesterol, but large-scale studies have proved it is no predictor of cardiovascular disease. Although it happens that Mrs Lowe had both arcus senilis and heart disease.

Finally, I turned to her notes. They completed the picture. *Busy lady, heart problems controlled by medication, often out and about and only very recently showed signs of forgetfulness. Flew to France to stay with son two years ago, met up with friends regularly, activity a bit curtailed by arthritis recently but still very sociable.*

Here, then, was Doreen Lowe. Not a totally healthy eighty-six-year-old, but a woman who was still thriving in old age. So, why was she here in the mortuary?

She was at home in her flat one evening when – and it is not clear how they entered – she was suddenly confronted by three young men. No one knows exactly what happened. Certainly, there was verbal abuse and some nasty threats. Certainly, Mrs Lowe responded robustly. She was persuaded to give them her purse, and that seems to have been enough for them because they then ran from the flat without taking anything further and apparently without touching Mrs Lowe. There were certainly no bruises on her body which could not be easily explained by subsequent attempts at resuscitation.

Mrs Lowe, showing great presence of mind after her ordeal, immediately dialled 999. The police soon arrived, to find her sitting in a chair in a state of shock. She had told the call handler what had happened but was unable to tell the police more before she collapsed. All attempts to revive her failed.

No doubt adrenaline had helped give her the strength to phone the police and tell the call handler in detail what had happened, to describe the intruders and even supply the name that one of the men had called another. As a result, the three were caught trying to enter another flat nearby with Mrs Lowe's purse still on them. They were immediately arrested. When it became clear that Mrs Lowe could not be revived, they were charged with her murder.

They insisted that they had not even touched her. That she had rapidly struck a bargain with them to hand over her purse if they would just go away, and they had agreed and left. Plus, how were they to know that she was about to drop down dead?

By eighty-six, many of our muscles must atrophy. Because, for all sorts of reasons (and the main one is arthritic pain), we don't use them as much as we once did. We may weigh less and sleep more and exercise little, so muscles lose bulk and the vigorous red of a robust muscle fades to something so pale it is almost pink.

Organs atrophy, too. Where the cells are still replenishing themselves, as in the liver, this may not be so marked. But after the death of heart muscle cells, for example, which are not replaced, the heart gets smaller. Perhaps this process can be delayed a little through exercise which raises the heart rate, but few eighty-six-year-olds use a rowing machine. And Mrs Lowe may never have exercised just for the sake of it. I daresay she had been busy with her job, her home, her children. No need to go to the gym. And, even if she had, those days were now far behind her. So the demands on her heart were few. Consequently, it had shrunken or atrophied, anyway, reduced in size by about two centimetres. This had created a problem for the coronary arteries which ran over it, supplying it with blood. They had a much smaller organ to cover and so they had to twist themselves like meandering rivers to fit into the diminished surface area available. Their white and yellow fibres swung this way and that over the soft, old heart.

In an eighty-six-year-old woman, the redundant reproductive system must also atrophy, this time from lack of use. The ovaries resemble discarded chewing gum. The womb has shrunk to something smaller than a walnut – a little larger if there have been two children or more. Nothing else will be asked of it and it has curled up into a firm, grey ball. Mrs Lowe had a benign polyp on the womb lining: she would not have known that, just as many women have no idea they have fibroids.

She had also, according to her notes, suffered from polymyalgia rheumatica, an autoimmune disease which causes great pain, very often in the shoulders, making it hard for some sufferers to raise their arms. I did not seek evidence of this, but I could easily find evidence for the congestive heart failure her doctor had reported. Her mitral valve was thickened and slightly calcified. Mrs Lowe would have experienced heart failure as leg swelling, tiredness and breathlessness because the heart could no longer pump blood efficiently enough around the body to meet her, no doubt low, demands on it.

And Doreen Lowe's heart problems did not stop there. She had severe atheroma in her right coronary artery. From scarring of the heart wall, I could see that there had been a small heart attack at least a year or so ago. I also identified mild diverticular disease in her large bowel and a cyst on her liver.

That is quite a list of major and minor health problems, and its length is not unusual in the very old. But which of these problems had actually caused Mrs Lowe's death after her terrifying brush with the intruders?

The fact is that Doreen Lowe could have died at any time because her heart disease was so severe, but she died immediately after this incident – actually within about ten minutes. The massive surge in adrenaline she experienced at the appearance of the intruders, followed by the dramatic increase in heart rate which her heart muscle was ill equipped to cope with, would have disturbed its rhythm to an unsustainable degree. Mrs Lowe had died as a direct result of the behaviour of the three lads and, of all the cases of such deaths I have written about here, this is the only one where the perpetrators were successfully prosecuted.

The key to prosecution is the very short space of time between the incident and the resulting death. Where this gap is so brief, it is much harder for the defence to argue that old age and not their client's action is the main cause of death, although if the gap had been more than ten minutes they certainly would have tried.

I was surprised to find myself feeling sorry for the perpetrators. Unlike all the other defendants in the cases here, they had not struck a single blow or laid a finger on the victim. They were all under eighteen, three lads out for a lark who either did not know or did not care how immensely upsetting their threats were to the vulnerable. Watching them standing in the defendants' box looking young and shocked, I could not help feeling that if someone had told them they would kill someone that evening, they would all have said they preferred to stay at home. But this is the risk for anyone when they choose to bully the very old: as the CPS keeps telling me, they must take their victims as they find them.

Last scene of all,
That ends this strange eventful history,
Is second childishness and mere oblivion;
Sans teeth, sans eyes, sans taste, sans everything.

21

We all want a long life, but does anyone want to live into senility? I know I don't.

In my youth, every old person dreaded having a stroke. This is no longer such a leading cause of death in the elderly, but it is still a significant cause of mental and physical impairment. A stroke can be a major event which results in a sudden and shocking disturbance to brain function. About half are ultimately fatal and, of those who survive, only 10 per cent of patients return to their previous normality.

In some ways, strokes can be similar to heart attacks: generally, they are caused by a blockage which kills cells in an area of a vital organ by preventing blood flow to it. Only, this time, the vital organ is the brain.

The blockage can take various forms. A blood clot. A piece of plaque or atheroma that breaks free and is carried along in the bloodstream, stopping when it is as large as the vessel carrying it. Or there can be a bleed into the brain when a tiny bubble blowing out through a weak area of an artery wall, an aneurysm, actually bursts – often because it has been battered by high blood pressure.

It can be easier at post-mortem to see strokes caused by a ruptured blood vessel than by a blocked one. Brain cells downstream of a blockage turn pale and soft after about a week. If the patient has survived the stroke, the tissue, starved of oxygen and blood, disintegrates. Holes, cracks and crevices appear. Where a stroke has been very severe, I may even find that half of the brain has collapsed, creating a disturbing asymmetry.

A stroke which has involved blood leakage looks different. The stain of the residual blood – brown, yellow, gold – will never go away.

A great risk factor for strokes, then, is high blood pressure. So are cigarette smoking, diabetes, alcohol consumption, a high-fat diet, lack of exercise, stress and, inevitably, genes. I fear some of these risks are present in my own life. If a doctor like me performs so poorly, despite full knowledge of the effects of his behaviour on his body, and despite living in luxurious circumstances compared with millions, what chance do those living in poverty have of defeating the monster? Poverty is the risk factor I didn't mention. Its link with heart disease and stroke is one for the epidemiologist, not the pathologist. But, statistically, that link exists.

Nowadays, the old do not fear stroke so much as they used to. They dread something else more. Dementia is currently the nation's biggest killer by a long way. Strokes and dementia are certainly not the same thing. Strokes may lead to dementia but, far from being a sudden, major event, dementia is a chronic condition and can have many causes.

Classically, it results first in the loss of short-term memory. This is usually followed by some loss of language skills, and then impaired decision-making. As the descent continues, it may be accompanied by anxiety. When there is a realization that this process is underway, that it is degenerative and that there is no intervention that effectively halts it, depression may follow. Later on, as the disease advances, the patient is no longer burdened with self-awareness. Those soundings we have taken all our lives from those around us, which help to regulate our behaviours and responses, are no longer available to us. We are left in a void with our core self. As memory is lost, the daughter is assumed to be the sister, then the mother and finally a stranger.

Gradually we unlearn all our parents taught us. How to talk. Clean our teeth. Dress in the morning. Walk. When all higher function is gone, the neurons in the more ancient part of our brain start to die. We can no longer sit up unaided or turn over in bed, and it is not the ageing body that prevents this but the ageing brain. We lose the ability to chew food. Even when food is liquidized, we cannot always swallow without choking.

Finally, immobilized, we may see but make no sense of sight. We can hear but, apart perhaps from music, the sounds are meaningless. We can touch soft things or feel the sun on the face or smell sweet perfume and, hopefully, experience some pleasure, but we can neither define nor recognize nor recall the sensory experience. We lose any memory of the recent past, initially, perhaps, retaining much from the distant past; we lose any knowledge of the future, and we may experience even the here and now at an isolating distance. If cardiovascular problems have contributed to dementia, then they may eventually cause death. But the most likely release is bronchopneumonia, which takes the enfeebled, undernourished and immobilized dementia sufferer with kindness.

The senile brain is distinctive. First, because it is small. In old age, we have lost a lot of brain cells and there can be quite a space between the skull's layers of inner lining and the surface of the shrunken brain. There is nothing much to stop it from wobbling around inside this cavity except for some scraps of haphazardly and loosely woven linen which, on closer inspection, looks more like a multitude of miniature stalactites. These are the tiny bridging veins and, now that the brain has shrunk, they must stretch across not a mere gap between skull lining and brain but a wide abyss. They are fragile with age and stretching far further than they used to. Therefore, they are vulnerable. How easy it is, for instance after a minor fall, for the shrunken brain to tear the tiny vessels when it moves inside the skull. Of course, they bleed. Here is a subdural haemorrhage.

Curiously, the very space that makes bleeding more likely can also ease its pain. It gives the leaking blood somewhere to go. A subdural haemorrhage for most of us is terrible, because the blood can create unbearable pressure in a very tight space. But, in the aged body, the blood can simply pool in the cavities created by the brain's shrinkage. The haemorrhage may even be unnoticed. At post-mortem, I might find a yellow-brown stain telling me that here, hiding, is the ghost of an old brain haemorrhage which caused so few noticeable symptoms in someone already suffering from dementia that it was never investigated.

Where else am I likely to encounter subdural haemorrhages? At the other end of life, in the brains of babies who have been cruelly shaken. But the end results are very different. For the old, a few, perhaps confused, years may lie ahead after such a haemorrhage. For the shaken baby, the result is often death or a long lifetime of persistent brain damage.

The senile brain, as well as being distinctively small, has a surface that is distinctively different. Those beautiful Alpine mountains and ravines of youth? We're still in the Alps, but we're lower down now, where the rivers have carved out wide, open valleys. It has been many years since the two sides of the valley have touched.

Cutting a cross-section shows just how wide the valleys are and reveals some more gaps. Internally, the brain has four great spaces, the ventricles and, when brain tissue is lost, these spaces slowly enlarge as their walls collapse away. Since the sterile fluid that surrounds the brain, the cerebrospinal fluid, is made inside the ventricles, this immediately fills the widening spaces. So now the ventricles look like some underground cave system: massive caverns, all full of liquid.

As senility increases, white matter, the wiring of the brain, diminishes. Anywhere in the brain, but perhaps especially around the ancient central ganglia, there may be areas full of tiny holes. Like the ruins left by an ancient civilization, these holes show where there were once great bundles of functioning neurons. And now the holes are filled with fluid.

So are changes to the brain not just normal but inevitable? Some diminution in brain tissue must occur, but genes and various lifestyle factors can modify this. It is important to come to terms with the fact that some brain cells are gradually lost as we age and, on the whole, we do not make new neurons. *On the whole.* The good news is that in recent years studies have indicated that cells are created in certain parts of the brain throughout life.

The hippocampus is small and hidden. It is named for its shape, which is rather like a seahorse. It is responsible for processing memory before storing that memory elsewhere and then accessing the memory when required. It helps, therefore, with navigation – without it, you would never find your way home. It also connects emotions or senses with memories. 'No sooner,' wrote Proust on drinking tea and eating a madeleine, 'had the warm liquid and crumbs touched my palate than I shuddered . . . and experienced an exquisite pleasure of the senses.' The pleasure came not from his immediate environment but the access he had gained through taste to a memory of childhood tea and madeleines with his aunt. That is the most famous example of the hippocampus hard at work.

Losing the way home and failing to reach elusive memories, let alone store new ones, are indicators of dementia, so a hippocampus that creates new brain cells is something we must surely all desire. Recent studies seem to show that we may be able to achieve this by exercising. All our lives. Including when we are old. The baseline here is the assumption that the hippocampus, in the elderly who show no signs of dementia, can shrink by 1 or 2 per cent in a year. However, after one year of aerobic exercise intervention, the hippocampi of participants in an Italian study actually increased in size by 2 per cent. Significant improvements in memory were noted after just three months. Other studies seem to confirm this by correlating higher fitness with a lower rate of cognitive decline and a decreased risk of dementia. So exercise does seem to spare brain volume a little.

The authors of the Italian report admit that so far there is a lot we don't know about the hippocampus, but they conclude:

Given the projected increase in the number of adults surviving to advanced age, and the staggering costs of caring for older individuals who suffer from neurological decline and mood disorders, physical activity may represent a simple, but effective and low-cost therapeutic intervention to improve neurocognitive and emotional functions. Furthermore, physical activity is accessible to most adults and is not plagued by the intolerable side effects often found with pharmaceutical treatments.

We used to be allowed to give as cause of death: Old Age. Forgetfulness and some physical impairment were accepted then and considered normal ageing. But, during my career, dementia has arrived to take over where old age stopped. Previously, the word 'dementia' had been used to describe patients who lost function or cognitive skills too early in life. This century's apparently massive leap in the numbers suffering dementia is not just because we are living longer but perhaps because we consider death at any age too early now. And because we are keener on definitions and we like to make old age a disease rather than just another step in life. Or maybe calling dementia a disease is our first step on the long road to understanding – and therefore, hopefully, one day to prevention and/or treatment.

The *Lancet*'s 2020 dementia commission is a fascinating review of all evidence about the causes of dementia. It says that 50 million people worldwide have this condition and adds that, with our current levels of obesity, diabetes and physical inactivity, the prognosis for *Homo sapiens* is not good. You can conclude from this that obesity is cited as a major risk factor: other predictable factors include smoking (or being around those who smoke), drinking and, perhaps not so obviously, air pollution.

The commission stresses that it is never too early or too late to engage with dementia prevention: some of these factors actually start in childhood and often it is midlife behaviours which will help avoid ill health much later. So, once you reach the age of forty, keep your systolic blood pressure (that's the first number the monitor gives you) at, or preferably below, 130 mm Hg. High blood pressure puts vessels under great strain. The consequences of this are many and various throughout the body but, in the brain, tiny vessels may quite simply give way, causing localized damage and resulting death to the tissues they supply. It is no good simply taking your blood pressure in later life and congratulating yourself that it has lowered or that your weight has dropped: at this stage, these changes may be signs of ill health, whereas in midlife they are almost universally promising indicators.

It is also important to protect the ears from loud noise all your life. When you do not have a history of hearing problems, but your hearing starts to fail, be honest, admit it, and use an aid. The impact of hearing loss is very significant: there is a direct correlation between this and cognitive decline. The correlation is non-existent in those who wear hearing aids. No one is sure exactly why this is so, but the isolation and reduced stimulation associated with hearing loss is one likely explanation.

To avoid dementia, we should avoid head injuries, including when young. Of course, we try to do this. No one wants a car crash. But certain sports – for instance, boxing, wrestling, soccer, rugby, American football, ice hockey – increase the risk, particularly at professional level. Repeated blows to the head, for example when soccer players head the ball, are, we now know, likely to result in Chronic Traumatic Encephalopathy. This is a neurodegenerative condition which manifests similarly to Alzheimer's disease.

The commission says that midlife is a particularly bad time for a head trauma – but is there a good time? My idiotic fall from that ladder and subsequent concussion is classed only as a minor traumatic head injury, but it has apparently doubled my chances of developing dementia.

Education, from the earliest years and for as long as possible, is probably vital for brain health in much later life. This is important information for parents and governments and is demonstrated by low- and middle-income countries, where childhood education may have been limited for an older generation but their life expectancy has increased: dementia is rising dramatically in some such countries. And here in the UK, the educational disadvantage in their youth of today's older generation of women may be reflected in their higher rates of dementia. The importance of education seems to be that brain use builds up cognitive reserves and, in my view and that of many others, this should continue through life. It means that, even when your brain pathology starts to work against you, you may have the adaptability to maintain everyday functioning.

Various studies highlight the importance of sleep from midlife onwards. Risk of all kinds of dementia is increased in those who sleep less than five hours a night or more than ten. And finally, there is a possible new and unwelcome risk factor. We have no idea what the long-term effects of the Covid-19 pandemic may be, but there is speculation that the immune response it triggers can cause significant inflammation of the brain. This may result, for some patients, in difficulties with memory and cognition as the brain ages. It is interesting that, at the time of writing, dementia is the most common underlying condition given on death certificates where the main cause of death is Covid-19.

For those of us who dread the possible onset of this condition, the *Lancet* commission's report contains one ray of hope: their estimate is that 40 per cent of dementia cases are preventable.

22

We do not know how great the suffering is of the dementia patient. Once it has progressed past the sufferer's awareness of the condition, is it possible to live with some degree of contentment? All we know for sure is that the comparison between the diminished sufferer and the person the sufferer was before onset can cause profound unhappiness in others.

It is the patient's family and their fears and feelings which can now become as important to manage as the patient's needs. The legal cases I am involved in when the deceased is extremely old and vulnerable are nearly all brought following family complaints to the police. The usual charge: lack of care, or even manslaughter.

Here is an extract from a very upsetting statement I was given by one family after the death of their elderly father, Albert Cannington. Mr Cannington was diagnosed with cancer of the pancreas when he was admitted to his local district general hospital on 3 September. He was reported as being in good health and not in any immediate danger, and some chemotherapy was recommended.

His family lived in another part of the country and asked for his transfer there but were told this could only delay the chemotherapy. Mr Cannington remained where he was and his son made the long journey to visit him on 19 September. The following week, on his eighty-fifth birthday, which was 26 September, all his four children gathered at his bedside.

'He may have been thin but he was in good spirits. We'd been worried that he had dementia but he asked us all about our families and jobs. I told him he might move to a hospital nearer us after his chemotherapy and he was very happy about that. We were there for two hours and he did not complain of any pain.

'On October 5th, a nurse phoned to say that he had deteriorated and now was very poorly. I asked if that meant he was dying, explaining that the family is scattered over England and that all of us are at least 200 miles away. She said that she was breaking rules by telling me but that she thought he might have only a few days left to live.

'I phoned my brother and sisters and we all went straight there. We found Dad asleep in a cubicle and we did not wake him. We devised a rota so that one of us would always be there.

'On October 6th, we asked to see a doctor. She said that Dad had pancreatic cancer and was terminally ill. I said that he was chatting and sitting up and didn't seem to be dying. In fact, we'd found him strong and talkative and alert. He had been much worse than this in the past and always pulled through. But the doctor said: "Your father is often confused. He has stopped eating. He is losing weight rapidly. Soon he will go into a coma and not wake up."

'I asked if he could go on a drip but the doctor said no and said she did not want us to move him closer to the area where I live. My daughter went out and bought some fruit juice, milk and Complan and a feeding mug with a spout. Dad ate quite a lot of it and enjoyed it.

'However, he began to go into deep sleeps and he kept doing strange things, like grabbing things in the air which weren't there. The nurse said that this was caused by diamorphine.

'Over the next few days, Dad went to sleep, and the staff

kept telling us it was a coma and he was about to die. They agreed it was time for the last rites, and the priest came.

'But sometimes Dad would wake up screaming or crying: help me, help me! Once he thought there was a fire. Every time it happened, we could see how scared he was, and it was heartbreaking to watch.

'We were not at all pleased with the way Dad was being treated. Because, actually, he wasn't treated at all. His pulse was strong and so was his grip. So we were worrying about a pump attached to his stomach which kept putting diamorphine into him. We kept asking for a drip and they said no. And almost no doctor came near him.

'On October 9th, I phoned Dr Kaye, who is a family friend and a private doctor. I begged her to come and, when she arrived, she saw Dad's skin and said he was very dehydrated. The ward doctor told her that Dad had pancreatic cancer, and that his chest was full of cancer too and that he would die very shortly. They had never told us anything about his chest. The ward doctor said that there was no need to put Dad on a drip because the morphine meant that he could feel no pain. But Dr Kaye told him that hydration was a necessity of life, practically a human right, and she asked them to give him a drip. She thought that would help make him less distressed too.

'Dr Kaye asked if she could examine Dad, and the ward doctor agreed so Dr Kaye lifted the bed covers and we were all horrified to see that he was just a skeleton. It was so terrible. Then Dr Kaye showed us a large open sore on his left buttock. There was pus oozing from it. She said this was an infected pressure sore. It did not have a dressing.

'Later, Dr Kaye said: "I am very sorry to tell you that your father is being killed by the hospital with diamorphine."'

Mr Cannington was not put on a drip. Over the next few days, the family became angrier and angrier: nursing staff referred them to doctors and doctors agreed to meet them and then did not appear or rushed off after scarcely conversing. Dr Kaye telephoned a number of times and was promised a drip would be put in place, but none was. Finally, Mr Cannington's son found himself face to face with a locum to discuss the IV.

'He told us: "Your father is dying and more active treatment will just prolong his death." He said that the diamorphine would not hasten death. I said that we loved our dad and that he was a strong man, too strong to die. We all wanted him to live and we had been asking for a drip for eight days and we wanted him to have one.'

There were more confrontations and phone calls before Mr Cannington was put on a drip and, at the family's insistence, this did not just hydrate Mr Cannington but also included vitamins to nourish him. Soon, Dr Kaye made the long journey to the hospital once again. She told the family that their father was very ill. His breaths were highly erratic, a pattern known as Cheyne–Stokes breathing, which sometimes precedes death. The family pleaded with her to get their father out of that hospital and she found a place for Mr Cannington at a cancer centre in the area where both she and the eldest son lived. Arrangements were made to transfer the patient by private ambulance. The hospital was not happy and asked the family to sign a disclaimer. They warned that they did not think Mr Cannington would survive the journey.

'I told the doctor that if Dad stayed there then he would certainly die,' writes the son.

On 15 October, they set off, two family members in the

ambulance and more in the cars which followed it. On his arrival at the cancer centre, they were able to see Mr Cannington's pressure sores for the first time.

The son writes: 'It was truly shocking and made us all feel sick. There were sores on his shoulders, back, buttocks, thighs, leg, foot. Dr Kaye took on his care. It was a huge task but she restored his dignity and he stopped being scared all the time. She cared for him lovingly and tenderly. She was kind and compassionate. And she was respectful. She tended him for many hours and we will be grateful forever to her.'

Mr Cannington died on 29 October. At which point, he became a police case.

It is worth looking at this sad story from the point of view of others involved.

First, Dr Kaye. She was clearly a compassionate and experienced doctor. Her relationship with the family evidently made her very susceptible to their demands at a time of emotional turmoil, demands that were rooted in their concern for their father and for his perceived needs. As a doctor of the less ill, she had no specialist knowledge of how these needs change if the patient's survival is not expected, but she clearly helped the family immeasurably.

She received the extremely frail Mr Cannington after his long journey to the cancer centre and immediately agreed with the family that his diamorphine dose should be halved. Her notes say that he was given a nourishing drip, turned every two hours and his sores were dressed. He was also given oral fluids and antibiotics to treat his infections. A ripple mattress was used to increase his comfort and lessen the pressure on his sores.

He had a high fever which gradually subsided, and an uneven heartbeat for which drug treatment was prescribed.

Through all this, although unable to talk, he did engage with his family, squeezing their hands and nodding in response to them.

As death got nearer, Dr Kaye explained that Mr Cannington's kidneys were failing and that there was not much more she could do. Evidently, the family did finally accept death's inevitability when presented by this trusted doctor. Various doctors communicated with the local hospice, but the son was adamant that his father should die in his (the son's) home. Mr Cannington was moved for one last time on 26 October. Dr Kaye continued to attend him, with help from the district nurses. When Mr Cannington died, three days later, Dr Kaye felt she could not issue a death certificate but instead, in view of the family's concern about his treatment at the hospital, contacted the coroner, who contacted the police.

Let us hear now from the hospital. One can well imagine how busy staff, the absence of the relevant consultant for a long period (she was on extended leave) and the constant presence on the ward of an increasingly angry family must all have been creating some strain.

According to the medical notes, Mr Cannington was admitted with carcinoma of the pancreas.

It was thought that chemotherapy was a good palliative option, but this took so long to arrange that by 5 October the doctor decided it was really too late, so greatly had Mr Cannington's condition deteriorated. He was often confused and was not able to take tablets and so he was given a syringe driver that would administer diamorphine up to pre-set limits.

Perhaps at that stage the hospital feared relatives' criticism, as it seems they were on the defensive. In his notes, the doctor wrote: 'His family may ask whether earlier treatment would have avoided this deterioration. The answer is that I feel it would have occurred even if the treatment had been started.'

As Mr Cannington's condition worsened, the hospital increased his morphine dosage. On 10 October, a doctor wrote: 'Condition very poor, eyes open in response to verbal comments, but no verbal response. Severe buttock and sacral infected bed sores. In pain when moved. It is unethical to prolong existence with further measures.'

The next day came a confrontation with the family, who were demanding rehydration. The senior house officer wrote: 'I agree with Doctors Eddison and Giraud that further active management will do nothing to alter the prognosis and add nothing to the patient's comfort. Active intervention at this stage would be both unethical and an insult to Mr Cannington's dignity. I have also been contacted by a Dr Kaye who is apparently attempting to influence our management of this patient. This is also inappropriate and unethical and, unless senior staff direct otherwise, Mr Cannington's management will remain unaltered, with the exception of pain relief, which will be administered as and when required in the appropriate quantity.'

The notes continue in a more personal way.

'NB It has come to our knowledge that Mr Cannington's relatives have not really visited him until the last few days and the question arises of their feelings of guilt. Maybe this is a factor in their persistent harassment of medical and nursing staff at all hours of the day and night. I personally feel that it is our responsibility to maintain Mr Cannington's comfort and dignity and I refuse to sacrifice this in order to placate his relatives. I have discussed this with [a consultant] and she agrees.'

This encounter was also recorded by Mr Cannington's son: 'The doctor said that Dad had been in hospital for a few weeks and actually asked me why we had not been here before. I think he was implying that we don't care about our father. I was very upset and told him we live all over the UK and that, anyway, we had visited our father on his birthday.'

It is clear that, by now, the trust of both parties had gone, family and doctors. The relationship between them was deteriorating in line with Mr Cannington's sinking condition. The next day, Mr Cannington was so distressed by attempts to turn him that his diamorphine was increased again. Two days later, after more discussions with the family, the hospital finally, reluctantly, agreed to release him for the 200-mile journey to the cancer clinic nearer the eldest son's house.

How easy it is to see everyone's point of view in this case.

It is easy to see how the family was tormented by the slow and unpleasant death of a loved father, and how hard it was for them to watch him effectively starve: extreme weight loss may be normal for a cancer patient, but for families it is anything but normal and they can find it very upsetting. The Cannington family, not unusually, associated the patient's great thinness with lack of care – and those bed sores too.

It is easy to see why the hospital chose to keep increasing Mr Cannington's pain relief so that he could not feel the bed sores, allowing them to turn him in order to relieve them. But perhaps pragmatism – low staffing levels, for instance, and the ongoing absence of the consultant in charge – also played a part in this decision. Certainly, there seems, from the hospital notes, to have been no lack of commitment to Mr Cannington's care – they continued with their plan and were determined not to indulge his family.

The subject of feeding or hydrating the dying is a cultural, ethical and medical minefield. Hospices usually do not use artificial means to give fluids at the end of life. Patients whose bodies are closing down as they move towards death often feel little hunger or thirst and the policy for most end-of-life carers is to interfere with this process as minimally as possible. In fact, there is some evidence that giving the patient more to eat or drink than is really wanted may cause real discomfort. There are gentler methods – mouth swabs and sprays, for instance – to satisfy a small need for hydration without the interference of tubes or drips. Artificial feeding this way can unnecessarily prolong life, just when the patient is quietly moving towards death. Also, the administration of artificial fluids has been linked in some studies to the more likely onset of terminal restlessness. This is a form of agitation which some patients can experience as the end nears and it requires calm and reassuring management – of both the patient and the devastated family.

Hospices have a thorough working knowledge of excellent end-of-life management, while it is generally the role of hospitals to prolong life. It was in line with hospice practice that the hospital decided not to rehydrate Mr Cannington. Perhaps, by hospice standards, they did this rather early in the process. They clearly expected him to die before he did and predicting death is unquestionably a dangerous business. But perhaps also his death might have occurred when anticipated without the extra nutrition and hydration Mr Cannington received from the drip his family demanded.

Yes, it is easy, from a distance, to see each party's point of view, but one of the key problems in this case is that no one could see Mr Cannington's death from anyone else's point of view. And, of course, the patient was not in a position to express his own wishes.

In his statement to the police, the eldest son says: 'I believe that the hospital doctors and other staff disgracefully neglected my father and you only had to see his pressure sores to know that must be true.'

And then he went further.

'I believe the hospital doctors are responsible for my father's death. I think they made a deliberate decision to end my father's life. He was given much more diamorphine than he needed. I also believe he was intentionally dehydrated and that when they deprived him of liquid, they deprived him of a basic human need and right.'

In fact, it is not uncommon in these circumstances for relatives to believe that medical staff are hastening death or, worse, actually killing the dying patient. It is an accusation that goes hand in hand with families' denial. Many hospices have learned how to manage relatives at this very emotional time, when tension is almost unbearable and hearts are breaking. They explain early on how the patient cannot be restored to a former self with meals or drips, but they encourage relatives to meet patients' physical needs in other ways. Some hospices have found this is something they must discuss at length and repeat often, so hard is it for denying relatives to believe. But in this case, all such communication between the hospital and the family was missing.

Initially, a hospital pathologist carried out a post-mortem in the presence of the police. The police then brought the case to me. And so Mr Cannington arrived on my post-mortem table.

He was, as expected, a pitifully thin old man with dark bed sores as large as dinner plates. These were all on the back of his body: on the front, his arms, hands and some parts of his legs were covered in huge purple blotches. These are the sort of bruises found only in the very elderly. They are called senile purpura and, although they look like a result of violence, they can be caused by even the light touch of routine care because skin is so very thin and inelastic.

I was soon able to find Mr Cannington's pancreatic cancer: a familiar hard, white crab nestling at the tail of the organ. But it was not his only area of significant ill health. The left ventricle's outlet to the aorta was severely narrowed by an aged aortic valve that had, over the years, calcified and could no longer function correctly. Consequently, his hardworking heart had enlarged to force blood through this ever-reducing gap. I found there was also significant atheroma in two more places, much lower down in the aorta, partially blocking the arteries to his kidneys. No wonder the hospital had completely ruled out operating on the tumour: with such arterial disease, Mr Cannington could not have survived any operation.

His liver was healthy but showed the changes associated with long-term heart failure. His bladder was infected. Resulting from both age and the blockage of his renal arteries by atheroma, his kidneys were small and very holey and miserable. They were no longer capable of doing their job. When I examined his lungs, I immediately saw pus ooze out of the airways and felt the frozen peas of bronchopneumonia.

Larger than these were the numerous firm lumps that I knew could mean only one thing. I examined them under a microscope. Yes, the hospital had been right. Mr Cannington's lungs were riddled with deposits of cancer which had metastasized from the pancreas.

I was, of course, expected to comment on the family's accusation that the hospital had deliberately hastened death by ramping up the diamorphine they gave Mr Cannington. The level described in his notes was quite high, but when someone is dying there really is no correct limit and cancers of the kind Mr Cannington had are known to be excruciatingly painful. I did not think his level of pain relief was designed to kill him: the art is to tread the fine line between alleviating pain and maintaining consciousness. Past a certain point, the latter is impossible, of course. However, the level prescribed is a clinical decision based on the exact needs of the patient on the day, and that is something a pathologist cannot judge in retrospect after death, and I declined to do so.

I could, however, deal with the other accusation, that of lack of care. The family was misguided about the hospital's failure to hydrate and provide nutrition to their father. The hospital's actions were entirely in step with current end-of-life guidelines, although this was very poorly communicated – leading to much more distress.

But what about those bed sores? They didn't kill him, but were they an indication of neglect? Mr Cannington had been admitted feeling very unwell. That – and his severely diseased arteries – suggested he had already been immobilized for some time, so he may have arrived on the ward with incipient bed sores. Or maybe not. Because, in a patient who is semi-conscious, suffering from arterial disease and unable to leave the bed, sores can appear and become established incredibly quickly, sometimes in just one day. Pressure sores may indicate lack of proper care. But, even with a fully staffed ward and constant nursing care, including frequent turning, their development cannot always be prevented and, once established, they are extremely hard to eradicate.

I gave as Mr Cannington's cause of death:

1a. Renal failure and bronchopneumonia
1b. Metastatic pancreatic carcinoma.

Had the family hoped that I would include: Lack of care? I could not do that. Only the coroner can make this decision, based on all the information. And he had correctly understood that Mr Cannington's death had natural causes. Despite some furious demands from the family, he did not hold an inquest but suggested that the son take up his complaints directly with the hospital. I was sure there were some grounds for complaint – but these were more about communication than medical issues. Hospitals must hold a thorough investigation into such concerns.

I have met many families in a state of bereavement over the years. I dreaded their horror and emotion when I first started to practise. How on earth could I manage that much grief? As soon as I witnessed it, I'd start to feel upset, too. Which of course was no good to them at all. Eventually, I learned that simply telling them the facts of their relative's death, explaining, reassuring, was the kindest thing I could do. I have met hundreds, if not thousands, of grieving families and they are all different and their grief takes different forms.

I did not meet the Canningtons. My information was restricted to the statements, the doctors' notes and Mr Cannington's body. My sense was that the father had been the lion of the family, a strong personality who had been regarded since childhood by his sons and daughters as invincible. And perhaps sometimes this had given rise to resentment.

Maybe all the family's actions arose from love and concern, as they claimed. Maybe not. They had certainly fought for every second of extra life for him that they could, although each second brought more pain. And that is why this case felt rather uncomfortable. I found myself unable to quell a small suspicion. That, in all this solicitous behaviour, there might have been some underlying cruelty. I felt that they almost certainly had increased their father's suffering. Had they, deep down, wanted to do this?

Of course, there was no way I could know what fault lines ran through this family. But I read through the notes again. I found, in the doctors' and nurses' earliest comments, and in the relatives' contact details, a record of a partner at the bedside, including her name. But Mr Cannington's partner then simply disappears from the story, mentioned by no one and certainly not by the son. That hinted at a pre-existing family division and perhaps a small battle for power over an increasingly powerless man? The family had been asking to move him far away right from the start; perhaps they wanted him moved far from the partner. Whatever battle took place, the partner evidently swiftly lost it.

It also seems significant that the hospital had to call the family in the first place to tell them that Mr Cannington was ill and had been admitted. I noted something that the staff also noticed. That, once informed, the Canningtons did not visit for two weeks and then came on consecutive weekends, one of which was their father's birthday. They were warned of his likely imminent death a month after he was admitted, and it was then that they set up their twenty-four-hour vigil at his bedside and began to lock horns with the doctors.

I remembered how my brother and sister and I had kept in touch with our father during his old and vulnerable years. None of us was overfond of our stepmother, but we were glad he had that relationship. Her presence did not deter me, since I lived the nearest, from sometimes getting up at 4 a.m. to make the round trip from London to Devon if we had any reason for concern. We all rang him often and regularly, and all three of his children took a keen and supportive interest in his health.

There is nothing special about us. But it was inconceivable that, had our father been admitted, we would have had no idea he was ill until informed by the hospital. And it was equally inconceivable that at least one and probably all of us would not then have visited him immediately. Or that we would have insisted his life was prolonged artificially when he was clearly near death. Or that we would have moved him during the end stage 200 miles. Or that, just before he died, one of us would have told doctors and the hospice that he must die in our own house and nowhere else.

I try not to measure others by my yardstick and probably it is unfair of me to harbour suspicions about the real feelings of this family towards their father. But here are the facts. Mr Cannington lay dying. He was still, helpless and semi-conscious, while anger and arguments raged around him. Although I believe that the time of death would not have been affected by this, it is not – must not – be how anyone should die.

Our understanding of a 'good' death has been challenged recently, and the challenge has come from the Covid-19 pandemic. Those who died in hospital in ICU must not be assumed to have had 'bad' deaths: they were well cared for, sedated, ventilated and unconscious when death came. This is, after all, a journey we are all destined to take alone one day, regardless of who sits at our bedside. But the suffering of these patients' relatives has been immense – as has that of the staff who cared for them, many making superhuman efforts to open channels of communication between the anxious, who could not be allowed in the hospital, and their dying loved ones.

This exclusion from the bedside has been terrible for relatives. They have been unable to hold the faltering hand or speak final words or offer comfort and love or just say good-bye. Dying may have been an entirely peaceful experience for patients, but Covid-19 has inevitably and unavoidably resulted in many 'bad' deaths for relatives. As Albert Cannington's family would wholeheartedly agree, the process of dying is not entirely about the departure of the patient: it is also about its impact on those left behind.

23

People often ask me what it's like to die. As if I know. As if anyone knows.

People who have died and been resuscitated describe very similar experiences whatever their religious beliefs, and these descriptions are of an event which is almost universally pleasant. There are possible physiological explanations for the beautiful lights, the reunions, the love renewed that survivors describe, but why look for one? Their descriptions confirm my own strong suspicions that dying is a process of almost exquisite sweetness. Whatever the manner of death, this process, once it begins, must be one of release.

So much of life is spent worrying, looking forwards in fear or backwards with resentment, game-playing, anticipating, regretting. So much time is spent on shopping and cooking and cleaning and maintenance and management as the shape of our families and our roles within them change. So many hours are spent arranging, planning, building, consolidating.

What a scramble it all is. And at the end, we let it go. The noise stops. With some sighs and perhaps a rattle, we release life. And once we realize that we have no choice, how can that release be anything less than enjoyable? Even when we fall asleep, we do not give in to such total relaxation as death brings: I don't think such a sense of release can possibly be achieved in life. And that applies whether we have a violent, untimely death, or long weeks of quiet preparation in a hospital bed.

It is a crime writer's fallacy that the faces of the dead reveal horror or shock or fear. They don't. No matter how death has occurred, the faces of the dead show quiet, peaceful repose. Let's remember that death is a process and not a sudden event. There is a moment of change, but the process can take minutes. The cells die gradually as the system winds down. Perhaps there is the sense of slowly relaxing into a warm bath.

I hope I have time to feel joy as I go. As I get older and worry less about death, I realize more and more what a wonderful experience life has been. Yes, all of it, the good and the bad, the fears and the happiness, the mistakes and the triumphs. Even the pain and the loss. Of course, there is the uplifting beauty of moors and mountains and lakes and oceans, but even the quotidian can dazzle me now with its beauty. I had no idea when I used to catch the bus to work in Tooting on a rainy morning that I would one day remember with pleasure the smell of wet raincoats, the clatter of feet on the stairs, the double ding of the bell as the bus slowed, the bright umbrellas threading their way outside, colours muted by the misted windows . . . I remember all these mundane details with an intensity I did not experience at the time. And I now recognize in them a beauty I could not see then.

I see the same beauty in my family and in those I love. And each time I take off in a small aeroplane and hear flight's silence, see the earth stretching to the horizon, bank and then watch the world rise up, I recognize that here is an exquisite painting with a detail and intensity no artist could reproduce. And I experience that beauty physically and mentally. This immersion in life's superlatives brings a joy which must vanquish all fear of death.

In this book you have read of death through homicide,

suicide, love, cruelty, madness and bad luck ... that is the world of the forensic pathologist. But death for most of us is not that way. Like my own father's, it takes place quietly, in the knowledge that life has been worth living and that we have been loved. I'd like to die in a chair reading a book, but one thing I know is that I really don't want to be asleep. In case I miss what may just be life's most wonderful experience.

Acknowledgements

There are many people who have influenced my life, and so this book. Mentioning some and not others is invidious, however, I'd like to specifically recall here my first mentor and teacher in forensic pathology at St George's Hospital Medical School. Dr Rufus Crompton sadly died from Covid while this book was being written.

Throughout my career, so many colleagues – crime scene investigators, forensic scientists, toxicologists, police officers, lawyers and coroners – from all around the UK and indeed the world have helped and guided me. They have done so on many occasions and in many ways. My whole-hearted thanks are always with you all for your friendship, knowledge, honesty, care and support. And for steering me around the odd pothole!

However, a book doesn't just appear, both it and the author need to be nurtured and supported, and I cannot fault the team at Michael Joseph who have cherished and helped me every step of the way with this project. Their methods involved a mixture of threats, love, cajoling and simple support, and my special thanks go to Rowland White, Ruth Atkins, Sarah Day, Laura Nicol and Sriya Varadharajan. And, of course, to Mark Lucas, ably assisted by Niamh O'Grady. Without them, I would probably still be drifting around, hoping that words and paper would magically unite to make something interesting.

Then my family, now scattered over the UK and indeed the world, always guaranteed to keep me in my place by producing a crisis just when I'm in the middle of a drama. What would I do without you all, who still contrive in so many ways to keep me 'young'? Chris and Anna, I really was young when you arrived in this world. And you have furnished my life with joy in more ways than I can count and, yes, you have taught me a lot too. You have both offered invaluable advice during the writing of this book: how could I have guessed all those years ago that one day I would rely on your wisdom and compassion? And my thanks also to my three 'extras', Rachael, Sarah and Lydia, who have each added so much extra to my life in so many different ways.

Into my own home now, where I'm fortunate to still have my constant companions and personal trainers Archie and Bertie, those faithful Jack Russells, always beside me as I write. They have heard my stories so many times that they may appear to be asleep but, whenever I move, they are at my heel. And finally, here is my lovely lady and wonderful wife, Linda, who truly saved my life one day when a swarm of bees, a broken ladder and gravity conspired to try to take it from me. How can I ever thank you enough for joining me on this wonderful journey?